MEDICAL PHYSIOLOGY

David Applin

SHREWSBURY COLLEGE LIBRARY		
INV. N. L174368	DATE	16/1/01
ORD. N. 33377	DATE	16/2/01
ACC. 034120		
CLASS. 612 APP		
PRICE £13-35	CHECKED	

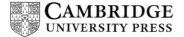

CAMBRIDGE
UNIVERSITY PRESS

SHREWSBURY COLLEGE
LONDON RD. LRC

PUBLISHED BY THE PRESS SYNDICATE OF THE UNIVERSITY OF CAMBRIDGE
The Pitt Building, Trumpington Street, Cambridge CB2 1RP, United Kingdom

CAMBRIDGE UNIVERSITY PRESS
The Edinburgh Building, Cambridge CB2 2RU, United Kingdom
40 West 20th Street, New York, NY 10011–4211, USA
10 Stamford Road, Oakleigh, Melbourne 3166, Australia

© Cambridge University Press 1997

First published 1997

Printed in the United Kingdom at the University Press, Cambridge

Typeset in Palatino 9.5pt

A catalogue record for this book is available from the British Library

ISBN 0 521 55661 9 paperback

Design by Hart McLeod, Cambridge

Cover photo: Science Photo Library

Notice to teachers
It is illegal to reproduce any part of this work in material form (including
photocopying and electronic storage) except under the following circumstances:
(i)   where you are abiding by a licence granted to your school or institution
       by the Copyright Licensing Agency;
(ii)   where no such licence exists, or where you wish to exceed the terms of a
       licence, and you have gained the written permission of Cambridge
       University Press;
(iii) where you are allowed to reproduce without permission under the
       provisions of Chapter 3 of the Copyright, Designs and Patents Act 1988.

Author's acknowledgements
It is a pleasure to acknowledge colleagues whose advice contributed to my
writing of *Medical Physiology*. In particular, I am indebted to the Reverend
Dr Michael Reiss who, as series editor, read the whole of the manuscript, and
to the Master and Fellows of Corpus Christi College, Cambridge, whose
hospitality during tenure of a Fellow Commonership provided the opportunity
for the work to progress. Finally the unstinting support of my family helped
ensure a successful conclusion to the project.

The publisher would like to thank the following for permission to reproduce photographs:
Wellcome Institute (1.1a,b); *Punch* (1.1c); Hans-Ulrich Osterwalder/SPL (1.2); Institut
Pasteur/CNRI/SPL (1.4); Richard T. Nowitz/SPL (1.8); National Medical Slide Bank (6.3);
Dr R. Dourmashkin/SPL (7.1); Manfred Kage/SPL (7.4); Hattie Young/SPL (7.6); Emily Bailey (9.4);
Addenbrooke's Hospital/SPL (9.5, 11.1); SPL (10.4); Cellmark Diagnostics (11.6); Will & Dennis
McIntyre/SPL (12.2).

Contents

What is disease?

Disease and good health are two sides of the same coin – how well we feel. A healthy person feels well because all parts of the body are working efficiently. Disease disrupts normal bodily functions and makes a person feel ill. A feeling of wellness is not just the absence of illness. Wellness includes mental health as well as bodily health – both are part of the equation defining good health.

The human body is an ideal environment for a range of organisms that cause different diseases. **Bacteria** are blamed for most human ailments, but **viruses** are also important disease-causing agents. **Protists, fungi** and different animal **parasites** also cause disease as a result of their activities inside our bodies.

Disease-causing organisms are called **pathogens**. Diseases are said to be **infectious (communicable)** if the organisms can be passed from one person to another. Not all diseases are infectious. Many **non-infectious** diseases develop because the body is not working properly. Increasing age and the way we treat our bodies affect the onset of non-infectious diseases. Many disorders can be avoided or at least delayed by changing our life-style.

1.1 Infectious diseases

During the nineteenth century the population of Britain more than trebled. People in search of work flocked to the cities, which were growing fast in the wake of the Industrial Revolution. London was typical of the times. With no proper means of waste disposal or sanitation, London's teeming population piled household rubbish and excrement outside the home. Water that was safe to drink was virtually unobtainable. Wells were contaminated by the filthy water draining from the streets; and the Thames, which was also a source of drinking water, was grossly polluted by raw sewage from most of the city. The insanitary conditions were ideal for the spread of infectious diseases.

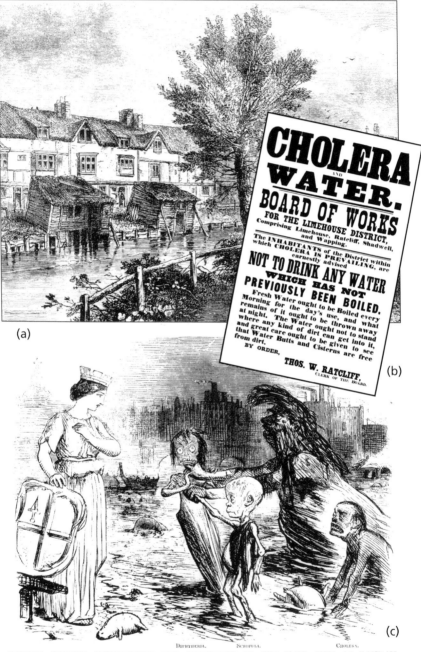

(a)

(b)

(c)

FATHER THAMES INTRODUCING HIS OFFSPRING TO THE FAIR CITY OF LONDON.
(A Design for a Fresco in the New Houses of Parliament.)

Figure 1.1 (*a*) Old houses in London Street, Dockhead: water supply and sewage disposal; (*b*) 1866 poster warning people living in the Limehouse district of London that the cholera epidemic was being spread by drinking unboiled water; (*c*) Cartoon from *Punch* satirising the polluted River Thames.

Cholera

Figure 1.1 shows a cartoon typical of the time. Images of disease were among many that cartoonists used to draw attention to the government's failure to safeguard public health. Though not at all clear about the true causes of disease, people realised that the Thames was a danger to health. For example, the poster in figure 1.1 links the spread of **cholera** to contaminated drinking water. We now know that cholera is carried in water contaminated with sewage, and is also transferred to food by flies. The image of slum housing in figure 1.1 shows why diseases like cholera spread so rapidly among the people of London and other major cities.

Cholera is caused by the bacterium *Vibrio cholerae* (figure 1.2). It results in a particularly violent form of diarrhoea due to the production of bacterial toxin in the intestine. Symptoms include vomiting and passing large amounts of liquid faeces. Loss of salts from the body causes severe cramps in the limbs and, unless treated, the patient can die within 24 hours from the effects of dehydration. In the nineteenth century there was no effective treatment and the death rate was very high. Today the disease is treated with the antibiotic **tetracycline** and fluids lost from the body are replaced, usually by **oral rehydration therapy** (see page 71).

In Britain and other developed countries, the provision of adequate drainage and sewage systems and the availability of a safe water supply have eliminated cholera (and other water-borne diseases). However, any large gathering of people (e.g. refugee camps), where sanitary arrangements may be rudimentary, remain at risk from outbreaks of the disease if drinking water is contaminated. Proper sewage treatment and chlorination of water supplies are the two most effective preventative measures.

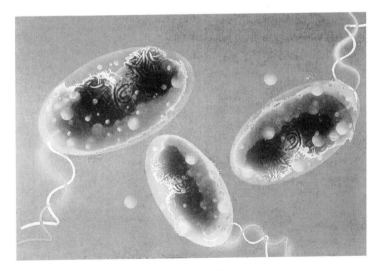

Figure 1.2 Scanning electron micrograph of *Vibrio cholerae.*

Tuberculosis

Scrofula is the old-fashioned name for a type of **tuberculosis (TB)**. The disease affects the lymph nodes (page 22), especially those in the neck. Symptoms include swelling of the glands and the development of abscesses. TB may also affect other organs, but the most common form is **pulmonary TB**, which attacks the lungs. The causative bacterium is *Mycobacterium tuberculosis*, which usually passes from person to person in droplets of moisture. Overcrowded living conditions such as those illustrated in figure 1.1 provide the long-term environment for the infection to gain a foothold and spread. A strain of TB affecting cattle can transfer to their milk and infect people drinking it. In Britain, pasteurisation of milk kills the bacterium, but worldwide, unpasteurised milk is a common source of the disease.

Pulmonary TB occurs in two phases:

- *Primary phase* – infections occur in different parts of the body and the victim may develop a dry cough that lasts for 3–4 months. A dormant phase follows which may last for several years.
- *Secondary phase* – increasing age and/or poor health may activate the causative bacterium, which usually attacks the lungs. Violent, frequent coughing brings up phlegm which may be tinged with blood. These are the symptoms of **consumption**.

Figure 1.3 shows the death rates from pulmonary TB since 1838. The reduction in overcrowding at home, improvements in hygiene and diet, and the development of antibiotics and an effective, safe vaccine (page 30) have reduced mortality dramatically. However, each year 6000 new

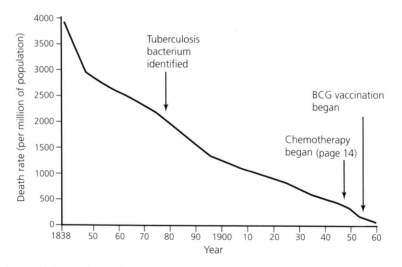

Figure 1.3 Death rate from pulmonary tuberculosis, 1838–1960. (Modified after Taylor D. (1989) *Human Physical Health*, Cambridge University Press.)

cases are reported in Britain, and worldwide the disease is estimated to kill between one and two million people a year.

How bacteria cause disease

Most types of bacteria are beneficial. What is it that gives a few types the capacity to cause disease?

- *Entry*: bacteria usually invade the body through the mucus-covered cells lining the gaseous exchange system, intestine, urinary system and genital ducts. To prevent their removal, bacteria produce substances called **adhesins** which link with receptors on the host cells. Bacteria can gain direct entry to the body where the skin is broken.

- *Penetration*: most bacteria must penetrate mucous surfaces to cause disease, although cholera bacteria need not. Dysentery bacteria (*Shigella* spp.), for example, produce cell surface proteins which promote the uptake of bacteria by the cells of the intestine.

- *Growth*: with the exception of iron, we know little about the nutrient requirements for the growth of bacteria within host tissues. In the case of iron, some bacteria excrete small molecules called **siderophores** which bind with iron. Receptors on the bacterial cell surface then recapture the iron-siderophore combination.

- *Interference*: the surfaces of bacteria are covered with substances that inhibit the action of the host's immune response (chapter 2). Many of the surface substances disguise other bacterial compounds which would otherwise act as **antigens** (page 22), triggering attack by the host's antibodies or granulocytes (page 25).

- *Damage*: toxins and effects on the immune response are the major sources of bacterial damage causing illness. Bacterial toxins are powerful poisons with dramatic effects. For example, the diphtheria bacterium produces a toxin that prevents protein synthesis in the host's cells. The toxin molecule is in two parts – one part is responsible for the toxicity and the other promotes uptake of the molecule by the **host cell**. The toxic component causes a swollen throat and massive internal bleeding. The damage caused by tuberculosis is due to the body's immune response to the bacteria causing the disease. **Granulocytes** (page 26) accumulate at sites of infection and release enzymes which break down lung cells. The damage can be seen on X-rays.

AIDS

AIDS stands for **acquired immune deficiency syndrome**. It is caused by the **human immunodeficiency virus (HIV)** (figure 1.4) which attacks the **T-helper** cells of the immune system (page 25). T-helper cells help protect the body against disease, so infection by HIV weakens the body's defences. People infected with HIV (*acquired*) do not suffer and die from the effects of the virus itself, but from the different infections (*syndrome*) which gain a foothold after HIV has destroyed sufficient numbers of T-helper cells (*immune deficiency*). The words in brackets highlight why this disease was given the name AIDS.

The virus attacks T-helper cells because it has surface protein molecules which match **receptor** proteins on the surface membrane of these cells. Once attached, the virus transfers its genetic material into the **host cell**, which becomes a factory for the production of new viruses under the direction of the genetic material from the infecting virus. Eventually each infected T-helper cell bursts open and releases thousands of new viruses which infect other T-helper cells. As the number of viruses increases, so does the number of T-helper cells destroyed, until the immune system is so weakened that the symptoms of AIDS set in.

After infection a short flu-like illness may occur. Following a period with no signs of illness, full-blown AIDS then develops in most patients. Infections that a healthy immune system would normally control take hold. Many HIV patients suffer from a rare form of skin cancer called **Kaposi's sarcoma**; other types of cancer, weight loss, diarrhoea, fever and deterioration of brain function are common. A rare type of pneumonia caused by the pathogen *Pneumocystis carinii* is a frequent cause of death.

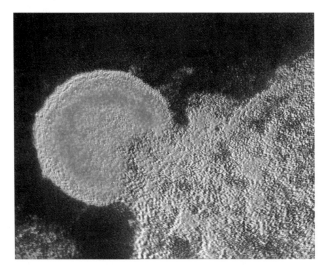

Figure 1.4 Transmission electron micrograph of HIV. The virus is budding from the surface of an infected T lymphocyte (a type of white blood cell).

A few HIV patients do not develop full-blown AIDS. A raised temperature and swollen lymph glands may develop but the onset of life-threatening diseases may be delayed indefinitely or at least for a long period of time. Quite why is not clear, but the condition is interesting to scientists searching for ways of helping the body fight HIV infection.

HIV is unique amongst the many viral infections affecting the human race in that it has a long **incubation period,** which is the time from when the virus infects the person to when the symptoms of AIDS develop. The incubation period may be up to 10 years. During this time, the person is HIV positive and able to pass on the virus to another person, often without knowing it.

The test for HIV infection depends on detecting antibodies (page 24) to HIV in blood samples. However, diseases such as tuberculosis and multiple sclerosis trigger the production of antibodies which can give a 'false-positive' result. Also, drug abusers, haemophiliacs (page 37) who require multiple blood transfusions and people exposed to a variety of infections all at once may give a positive result because the immune system is weakened, even though they are not infected with HIV.

Transmission

Transmission of HIV is usually by sexual contact, the communal use of contaminated syringes and needles by drug abusers and, early on in the history of the disease, by transfusion or infection of blood or blood products. Haemophiliacs who required regular injections of factor VIII (page 35) were particularly at risk. However, the developed countries introduced sterilisation and screening of donated blood for HIV infection (the procedures have been in place in Britain since 1985), and now the risk of HIV transmission from the use of blood and blood products is virtually non-existent (page 37). Sexual transmission of HIV between male homosexual partners often occurs during anal intercourse when the tissues lining the anal passage may be damaged following penetration of the penis and release of semen by the active partner. HIV is present in seminal fluid. Heterosexual transmission through vaginal intercourse is less common except when people have a large number of sexual partners and/or misuse drugs. Either partner may infect the other. HIV in secretions from the vaginal wall pass to the male via his penis; HIV in seminal fluid passes to the female via the lining of the vagina, cervix and uterus. In either sex the risk of infection is considerably increased where the genitalia are either ulcerated or abraded.

The communal use of contaminated syringes and needles by intravenous drug abusers remains a considerable problem. Sexual contac between drug addicts and other members of the public is also an important route for the spread of HIV infection. For example, female addicts, in particular, often turn to prostitution to finance the purchase of drugs.

Because HIV has a long incubation period, data on the progress of AIDS reflect patterns of HIV transmission several years ago. Figure 1.5 shows the progress of AIDS in England and Wales for different categories of people. Notice that homosexual men are at greatest risk, but that sex between men and women accounts for nearly 20% of cases in 1993 compared with under 10% in 1990. Successive governments have launched, with some success, advertising campaigns that highlight the threat from HIV infection through 'unsafe' sex and drug abuse. As people's patterns of behaviour change, then so too will the pattern of HIV transmission and the progress of AIDS.

Treatment and prevention

The search for ways of treating and preventing HIV infection is worldwide. A twin-track approach focuses research in the following areas:

- Developing drugs which deactivate HIV. Scientists aim to identify weak links in the virus's metabolism and develop drugs that break the chain of infection. The best known drug in use is **zidovudine** (sometimes called **AZT**). It stops HIV from replicating (reproducing) but can have harmful side effects. For example, patients taking AZT may develop anaemia (decrease in the number of red blood cells). Research continues in order to

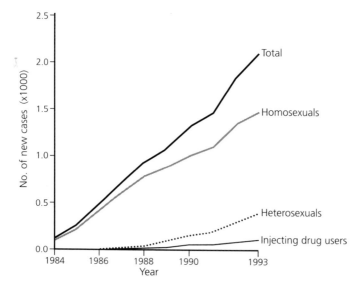

Figure 1.5 New cases of AIDS for different categories of population in England and Wales, 1984–93.

Source: PHLS Communicable Disease Surveillance Centre.

find drugs with which to attack different stages in the HIV life
cycle.

- Vaccine development. This offers the best hope of attacking HIV
  and preventing AIDS.

However, HIV poses a formidable challenge:

- The amino acid sequence of its protein envelope alters
  constantly. The amino acid sequences are the major antigens
  against which antibodies are produced (page 22).
- Because the virus transfers its genes into the host's T-helper
  cells, there are no viral antigens on the surface of the T-helper
  cells for antibodies to attack. The virus, therefore, is 'invisible'
  to the infected person's immune system. Moreover, the viral
  genes inside each host cell control the replication of new viruses
  which eventually escape to infect other host cells when the
  original host cell bursts open.
- It is a **retrovirus** and retroviral genes cause cancer. A vaccine,
  therefore, based on attenuated whole virus (page 30) could
  cause cancer.
- At first sight, production of antibodies that prevent HIV from
  attaching to T-helper cell surface receptor proteins seems,
  potentially, to be a powerful way to attack the virus. However,
  scientists' efforts have been frustrated because a second wave of
  antibodies is produced against the first, which attacks the T-
  helper cell surface receptors and destroys the T-helper cells.

While the search for new drugs and vaccines continues, taking precautions
is the most effective preventative measure against HIV infection:

- Using condoms during anal or vaginal intercourse provides a
  mechanical barrier to transmission of the virus.
- Provision of sterile needles and syringes reduces the risk of
  infection from shared 'equipment' among drug abusers.
- Screening donated blood for HIV antibodies and rejecting blood
  containing these antibodies reduces the risk to patients in need
  of transfusion. Heat treatment of blood plasma containing factor
  VIII kills HIV without destroying the factor VIII protein.
  Haemophiliacs who depend on injections of factor VIII (page
  35) are therefore protected. Genetic engineering also provides a
  safe source of factor VIII (page 37).

The social consequences of HIV infection and AIDS are profound. The
costs of research, patient care and counselling services for HIV positive
people, their families and friends are huge and detract from other areas
of research and medical care. Throughout history, the human race has been
afflicted with diseases that achieve a 'high profile' through their virulence,
their effects on people and the way that society responds to them. Think

of the bubonic plague in medieval times, small pox in the seventeenth and eighteenth centuries and, more recently, polio. HIV infection and AIDS could be another example of public attitudes affecting behaviours that put people at risk from infection, and where research will eventually provide the solution. Imagine the post-AIDS future. How do you think people will react when the threat of HIV infection is lifted?

Malaria

There are four species of the protist *Plasmodium* responsible for human **malaria**. The parasite infects liver cells and red blood cells. Once *Plasmodium* is in the bloodstream, flu-like symptoms are followed up to 30 days later by high fevers, chills and heavy sweating. The timing of attacks depends on the species of *Plasmodium*. *Plasmodium vivax*, the most common species, causes a mild form of malaria; figure 1.6 shows the development of symptoms. *Plasmodium falciparum* is the most dangerous. It may cause red blood cells to become sticky, blocking blood vessels to the brain, kidneys, intestines and lungs. Unless treated, the victim may die within a few days.

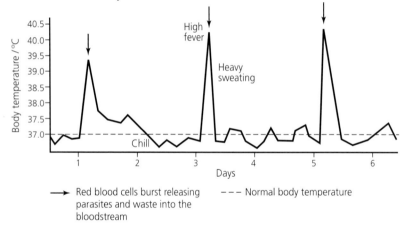

Figure 1.6 Changes in body temperature following infection by *Plasmodium vivax*.

About 30 different species of *Anopheles* mosquito worldwide are responsible for transmitting *Plasmodium* parasites to humans. Females need a blood meal as well as sugary liquids (e.g. nectar) before their eggs can develop. They are able to feed on most vertebrates (including humans). The female's pointed mouthparts pierce capillary blood vessels beneath the surface of the skin and take up blood like a hypodermic needle. If the person is already infected with *Plasmodium*, then the parasite is sucked up as well and passed on when the mosquito feeds on another person.

Geography

In Roman Britain the Thames Valley and the marshlands of East Anglia were ideal breeding grounds for malaria mosquitoes. The disease was common in the sixteenth century, when it was called the **ague**. Over the centuries land drainage, a cooler climate and better living conditions resulted in the eradication of malaria from Britain by the early 1900s. Today, cases reported in the UK are of people returning from visits abroad where the disease is endemic.

Figure 1.7 summarises the distribution of malaria. *Plasmodium* needs warmth to reproduce inside the mosquito, and the disease flourishes in the warmer regions of the world. Poorer countries are particularly vulnerable, as they are short of expert help and find it difficult to finance measures for treatment and prevention.

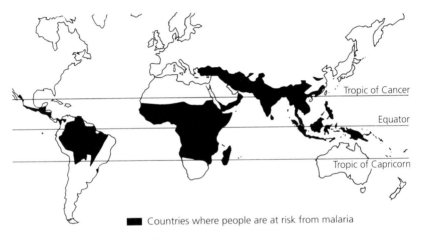

Countries where people are at risk from malaria

Figure 1.7 Worldwide distribution of malaria.

Life cycle

Since *Plasmodium* infects blood, feeding on blood makes female mosquitoes efficient **vectors** of the parasite. Unlike people, they are unaffected by it. Figure 1.8 shows the role of mosquitoes and people in the malarian life cycle.

Repeated invasions of red blood cells are tracked by the cycle of chills and fevers shown in figure 1.6. The victim's body temperature soars when the red cells burst releasing parasites into the bloodstream. Eventually, enormous numbers build up causing serious and sometimes fatal illness.

Treatment and prevention

Fighting malaria depends on destroying the adult mosquito vector and its aquatic juvenile stages, destroying the parasite, or preventing contact between the vector and people. Control measures are:

- *Draining* marshes, ponds and ditches, preventing the female mosquito from laying eggs, and the eggs developing into larvae. It is, however, too expensive, and indeed impossible, to drain all breeding areas.
- *Biological control* in the form of fish which eat mosquito larvae. This method is less successful with mosquitoes compared with some other examples of biological control. The best known biological control agent for malaria is the larvae-eating minnow *Gambusia affinis*, which has been introduced from the USA into many countries where malaria is endemic.
- *Insecticides* sprayed on the water's surface, killing mosquito larvae and pupae. Unfortunately other forms of wildlife are killed as well. Spraying persistent insecticides like DDT on the interior walls of houses kills adult mosquitoes resting on them but causes long-term damage to the environment.
- *Drugs* like quinine, chloroquinine and quinacrine, which prevent multiplication of the parasite in the red blood cells of the host, and paludrine, which inhibits the parasite's life cycle in

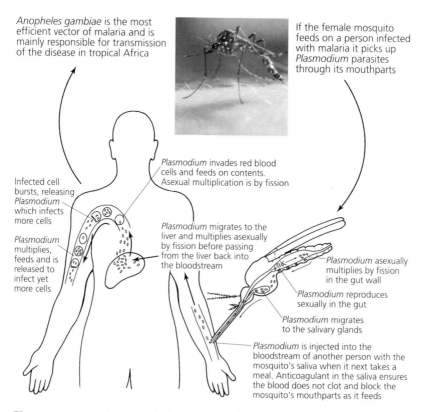

Anopheles gambiae is the most efficient vector of malaria and is mainly responsible for transmission of the disease in tropical Africa

If the female mosquito feeds on a person infected with malaria it picks up *Plasmodium* parasites through its mouthparts

Plasmodium invades red blood cells and feeds on contents. Asexual multiplication is by fission

Infected cell bursts, releasing *Plasmodium* which infects more cells

Plasmodium multiplies, feeds and is released to infect yet more cells

Plasmodium migrates to the liver and multiplies asexually by fission before passing from the liver back into the bloodstream

Plasmodium asexually multiplies by fission in the gut wall

Plasmodium reproduces sexually in the gut

Plasmodium migrates to the salivary glands

Plasmodium is injected into the bloodstream of another person with the mosquito's saliva when it next takes a meal. Anticoagulant in the saliva ensures the blood does not clot and block the mosquito's mouthparts as it feeds

Figure 1.8 Route for transmission of *Plasmodium* in malarian life cycle.

the mosquito. Over-use of drugs for the treatment of malaria has led to the development of resistant strains of *Plasmodium*. The **World Health Organisation (WHO)** recommends that new anti-malarial drugs should be used selectively to slow the spread of resistance.

- *Vaccines* which inhibit different stages in the parasite's life cycle.
- *Bed nets* soaked with insecticide to protect the resting person not only from mosquitoes but from other biting insects as well. The method is cheap and effective but makes sleeping conditions hotter. In Gambia, West Africa, bed nets soaked in insecticide have reduced the death rate from malaria by 70%. The aim is a country-wide scheme to protect people from mosquito bites.
- *Chemical repellants* like diethyl toluamide sprayed onto the skin and clothes to deter mosquitoes from landing on the body. However, their effect soon wears off, especially if the person is sweating heavily.

Quinine is the oldest drug used in the treatment of malaria. It was first isolated in 1820 from the cinchona tree which grows in the tropical rainforests of the Amazon, South America. People who live in the forests chew the bark of the tree to protect themselves from fever.

Natural immunity

In many parts of Africa people show partial immunity to malaria. The body produces antibodies in response to *Plasmodium* which prevent infection of the liver cells and red blood cells or destroy red blood cells already infected. Other immune responses have similar effects.

The unborn child of an infected mother is given some protection by maternal antibodies which cross the placenta before birth. This **passive immunity** (page 31) disappears 4–6 months after birth. However, if the child survives to reach the age of 5–6 years, then repeated infections result in **acquired immunity**, which gives a high level of protection.

Sickle-cell trait and malaria

Sickle-cell anaemia is caused by a **mutation** in the genes controlling synthesis of the blood pigment **haemoglobin**. The **codon** specifying the amino acid glutamate – GAG – mutates to GTG which specifies the amino acid valine. This substitution results in a drastic reduction in the oxygen-carrying capacity of haemoglobin. Individuals who inherit the sickle-cell allele from both parents (the **homozygous** condition) often fail to reach adulthood. Although the frequency of the sickle-cell allele is low in cooler, temperate countries, in parts of Africa and other warmer regions of the world it may be carried by up to 30% of the population. How does a potentially lethal allele persist at such high frequency? Part of the answer is that as the sickle-cell allele is recessive, its effect is masked if it is partnered with a normal allele. So, individuals who carry just one sickle-cell allele (the **heterozygous** condition called **sickle-cell trait**) show few if any of the symptoms of sickle-cell anaemia. In addition, the *Plasmodium* parasite causing malaria is unable to attack the carrier red blood cells as effectively as normal red blood cells. People who are heterozygous carriers therefore show greater resistance to malaria than individuals who are not, and are more likely to survive and have children. So the sickle-cell allele is inherited and persists from generation to generation because of its survival advantage in areas where **selection pressure** from the malaria parasite is high.

Are genetically engineered mosquitoes the future for malaria control? Some scientists think so. Ideas include equipping mosquitoes with genes that block development of the *Plasmodium* parasite inside the mosquito gut. However, overcoming the technical problems may take years, not least that of finding ways of inserting the 'foreign' genes for *Plasmodium* destruction into the mosquito **genotype** (page 133) and ensuring that they spread through the mosquito population. Critics think the scheme will fail because of the difficulties, and that meanwhile scarce resources are being diverted from research into other more promising methods of control. Who is right? The arguments highlight the difficulties of prioritising research, and identifying that which results in both scientific progress and practical benefits.

1.2 Fighting disease

With so many pathogens capable of infecting humans, why do most of us stay healthy most of the time? The body itself is the first line of defence. For example, the skin is an important barrier against infection. **Antiseptics** are chemicals that prevent microorganisms from multiplying. They can be used to clean the skin and stop microorganisms from becoming established. **Disinfectants** kill microorganisms. Stronger than antiseptics, they are not used on the skin but help to keep surfaces clean and free from microorganisms. For example, bleach (which contains calcium chlorate) is a strong disinfectant used to kill microorganisms that lurk in drains and lavatories.

The term **chemotherapy** describes treatments which use drugs to attack pathogens and other causes of disease. (There is more about drugs and the treatment of disease elsewhere in the book.) An important group of drugs are the **antibiotics**, e.g. tetracycline, which is used in the treatment of cholera (page 3). Thanks to antibiotics, the majority of bacterial diseases can now be cured. There are two sorts of antibiotic: those, like tetracycline, which prevent bacteria from multiplying, and those, like penicillin, which kill bacteria. Figure 1.9 shows how different antibiotics affect bacteria.

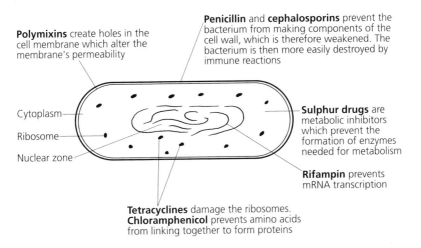

Polymixins create holes in the cell membrane which alter the membrane's permeability

Penicillin and **cephalosporins** prevent the bacterium from making components of the cell wall, which is therefore weakened. The bacterium is then more easily destroyed by immune reactions

Cytoplasm

Ribosome

Nuclear zone

Sulphur drugs are metabolic inhibitors which prevent the formation of enzymes needed for metabolism

Rifampin prevents mRNA transcription

Tetracyclines damage the ribosomes. **Chloramphenicol** prevents amino acids from linking together to form proteins

Figure 1.9   How different antibiotics affect bacteria.

Vaccines protect millions of people worldwide from serious diseases. Vaccine production, vaccination (immunisation) and the biology of the **immune response** are dealt with in chapters 2 and 12. Here we shall examine the social importance of vaccination, especially for children.

In Britain, children are vaccinated against diseases which used to cause many deaths. Table 1.1 shows the vaccination programme. The diseases listed are now rare but would soon increase if the number of people vaccinated fell to levels at which infections spread easily. The diseases listed in table 1.1 kill 3.5 million children annually in developing countries. However, governments recognise increasingly that vaccination programmes are effective methods of protecting people from life-threatening diseases. Various scientific and social breakthroughs are helping to increase the rate of vaccination:

- development of vaccines which 'keep' for longer, even in hot climates;
- increasing availability of refrigeration equipment for storing vaccines in developing countries;
- increasing numbers of health workers being trained to give vaccinations;
- governments taking measures to educate and inform parents of the benefits of vaccination.

Table 1.1. Recommended vaccination programme for children in Britain

Age/years	Disease	Programme	
0–1	Diphtheria Tetanus Whooping cough *Haemophilus influenzae* type B	} By injection	} 1 dose of each vaccine given at 2, 3 and 4 months
	Poliomyelitis	By mouth (oral vaccine)	
1–2	Measles Mumps Rubella (German measles)	} By injection	
3–5 (school entry)	Diphtheria Tetanus Poliomyelitis	} Booster injections	
13	Tuberculosis	By injection (BCG) following negative Heaf test	
10–14	Rubella	By injection for girls who have not been vaccinated previously	
15–19 (school-leavers)	Tetanus Poliomyelitis	By injection By mouth	

Worldwide, vaccines prevent about 800 000 deaths from infectious diseases each year. Developing countries are rapidly increasing their programmes to further reduce the number of deaths from diseases that can be prevented by vaccines.

1.3 Non-infectious diseases

In developing countries, 40% of all deaths are caused by infectious diseases, e.g. diarrhoea and measles, associated with inadequate medical services, poverty, poor housing and malnutrition. In developed countries where there are good medical services, relatively few people die from infectious diseases. Instead, diseases associated with life-style and old age – non-infectious diseases – are the major killers. We are living longer and can afford to smoke, drink too much alcohol and eat too much of the wrong sorts of food. Crippling diseases such as arthritis are associated with old age, and unhealthy life-styles are responsible for the onset of heart disease (chapter 4) and cancer – both leading causes of death in many developed countries.

Cancer

Cells divide when grown on dishes in a solution of all the substances they need to live. Normal cells spread until neighbouring cells touch each other, forming a layer over the bottom of the dish. At this point **contact inhibition** stops further division. **Cancer** cells are different. They continue to divide even when they are all touching. Piling up, they form a mass. In the body, masses of cancer cells are called **tumours**. By multiplying faster than normal cells, cancer cells destroy healthy tissue.

Cancer is not just one disease but about 200. The number of deaths each year from the nine commonest types of cancer in the UK, are given in table 1.2.

The transformation of normal cells into cancer cells occurs in stages, beginning with genes. Some genes switch on the processes that make cells divide; others slow down or stop cell division. If 'switching on' genes or 'stop' genes are damaged, or if 'stop' genes are missing, then cell division may run out of control, leading to cancer.

Table 1.2. Annual deaths in the UK from the most common forms of cancer. Cancers cause around 1 in 4 deaths in the UK

Cancer	Deaths
Lung	40126
Bowel	19391
Breast	14983
Stomach	9864
Prostate	9048
Pancreas	7074
Oesophagus	5868
Bladder	5512
Ovary	4489

If detected early, many cancers can be cured by surgery, chemotherapy and/or radiotherapy using a radioactive source. If left untreated, however, cancerous cells can break away from the original (**primary**) tumour, spread (a process called **metastasis**) and set up **secondary** growths elsewhere in the body, endangering the person's life.

New treatments for cancer are under development:

- Drugs that prevent division of cancer cells.
- Vaccines against cancer-causing viruses. For example, cattle suffer from papillomaviruses similar to the virus that causes cervical cancer in women. Scientists have developed an effective vaccine for the cattle virus and the race is on to develop the human equivalent.
- Replacement of faulty genes with healthy copies.

Meanwhile, successful treatment for cancer depends on early detection before the cancer can spread in the body.

Osteoporosis

Bone strength and density depends on the balance between the activities of two types of cell:

- **osteoblasts**, which secrete fibrils of the protein **collagen** in which **calcium** compounds are deposited;
- **osteoclasts**, which break down bone, releasing calcium into the blood.

The balance between the activities of osteoblasts and osteoclasts determines bone density. **Osteoporosis** develops when the activity of osteoclasts outstrips the activity of osteoblasts. Severe loss of calcium from the bones makes them porous and fragile, and more liable to break.

Osteoporosis is age-related. Women are particularly vulnerable because **oestrogen** affects the absorption of calcium ions (Ca^{2+}) from the intestine and therefore the availability of calcium to the bones. Production of the hormone drops dramatically after **menopause** (around the age of 40–50 years). **Hormone replacement therapy** (page 87) aims to prevent the onset of osteoporosis by maintaining oestrogen at pre-menopausal levels. Ideally, however, prevention begins in childhood. Exercise and an adequate intake of milk (a rich source of calcium) encourages sturdy bone formation.

Calcium supplements alone do not halt the progress of osteoporosis. Hormone replacement is necessary to ensure adequate absorption of calcium, and treatment with anti-inflammatory drugs damps the activity of the osteoclasts.

Arthritis

As we grow older, wear and tear on the joints may cause pain and even make it difficult to move freely. Pain in the joints is often called **arthritis**, but the word covers conditions ranging from degenerative joint disease to gout. For example, **rheumatoid arthritis** affects the joint surfaces. The cartilage that makes for the smooth, friction-free movement of joints is destroyed, possibly as a result of the body producing antibodies against itself. Diseases caused by disturbance of the body's immune system are called **auto-immune** diseases (page 22).

Osteoarthritis results when joint surfaces wear faster than they can be repaired. Quite why the cartilage breaks up more in some people than others is not clear, but if the joint is subjected to excessive strains and stresses, then the damage develops more quickly. Obesity or fractured joints make a person particularly vulnerable to the development of osteoarthritis, hips and knees being especially affected.

When the pain and stiffness reach a stage where walking even short distances is difficult, then the joints may be replaced. Replacement parts for diseased hip joints have been developed since the 1950s. Replacements are so effective that thousands of operations are performed each year. There are two components to a replacement hip joint: a ball and shaft made of stainless steel, and a high-density plastic cup into which the ball fits. Ball and cup are fixed into the bones with cold-setting acrylic cement.

1.4 Social consequences of ageing

Table 1.3 shows a medical success story and a developing social problem. Research is delivering new treatments, new drugs and better healthcare with the result that, on average, people can now expect to live longer than those of previous generations. Death rates are falling such that the average life span is increasing by about two years every decade. Not surprisingly, therefore, the population of the UK is ageing. One hundred years ago, 6% of the population were over the age of 65; today the figure is around 18%. Simple statistics highlight the impact of the changes:

- Between 1980 and 1990 doctors provided around 52 million extra prescriptions for medical items (drugs, appliances, etc.). Of these extra prescriptions around 95% were issued to the over-65s.
- Currently nearly half of all social security payments (amounting to around £39 billion) are made to the elderly.

The economic demands of an ageing population and society's ability to cope with its medical and social needs are major challenges now and for the future.

Table 1.3. UK life expectancy and number of people aged 65 and over

| Year | Expectation of life/years | | Number of people aged 65 and over/millions | Total number of people – all ages/millions |
	Male	Female		
1901	45.5	49.0	n/a	38.2
1931	57.5	61.6	n/a	46.0
1961	67.8	73.6	11.7	52.8
1971	68.8	75.0	13.2	55.9
1981	70.8	76.8	15.0	56.4
1991	73.2	78.7	15.7	57.8
2001*	75.4	80.6	15.7	59.7
2011*	76.8	81.9	16.6	61.3

*Projection
Source: based on figures from the Government Actuary's Department.

Research aims to lift the threat of diseases that commonly blight the lives of the elderly. These include osteoporosis, Alzheimer's disease (page 110), Parkinson's disease and breast cancer. Meanwhile, the current emphasis on healthy diets, not smoking, limiting alcohol intake and taking modest amounts of exercise improves the quality of life so that more years are spent in relatively good health. Increasingly, therefore, old age can be enjoyed rather than feared.

1.5 Rhythms of life

Changes in living processes often occur in rhythmic fashion. This means that organisms (including human beings) differ biochemically and physiologically at different times of day and night, and respond differently to the same stimulus depending on its timing. The effectiveness of drugs is a case in point. The times at which drugs are administered and the quantities given at the different times are critical. For example, proper timing of drug doses during chemotherapy for cancer can significantly improve the survival rate of patients. Therefore, understanding a patient's rhythms – their **chronobiology** – helps determine when treatment will be most effective.

Many physiological responses approximate to a 24-hour cycle, and for this reason they are called, **circadian rhythms**. It is well known, for example, that body temperature fluctuates by as much as 1°C during the course of 24 hours, reaching a low at around 4 a.m. and a peak at around 4 p.m. Excretion in the urine of potassium, sodium and calcium, and secretion of different hormones and enzymes, all vary according to the time of day. For example, production of **alcohol dehydrogenase** peaks in the late afternoon. The enzyme metabolises alcohol in the liver, and so alcohol tolerance is greatest at around 5 p.m. These and other physiological rhythms have been observed in many people on a normal sleep-wake cycle.

Not surprisingly, **shift** work disturbs the pattern of the body's activities. People who work night shifts and who sleep during the day often report feeling 'under the weather' after beginning the routine, until their physiological rhythms have had time to adjust. Pilots and passengers who fly from one time zone to another experience similar effects. Called **jet-lag**, the symptoms are a result of the desynchronisation of the body's functions with daily activity, and may persist for as long as a week after a long-distance flight.

In many instances, rhythmic changes are achieved by means of **biological clocks** located within the cells. These 'clocks' work independently of changes in the physical environment, which nevertheless serve to 'set' the clocks so that the physiological responses occur 'on time'. In the absence of environmental cues, the clocks, and the physiological responses they control, 'drift' but still persist. Renewed exposure to environmental cues 're-sets' the clocks, and their physiological responses return to the 'right time'.

T W O

Understanding the immune system

Immunology is the science concerned with the processes and mechanisms that establish specific immunity against the bacteria, viruses and many different substances that can harm the body. Together, these processes and mechanisms make up the **immune response.**

2.1 The specific immune response

Antigens are substances that can trigger an immune response. **Self antigens** are part of the membranes of our body cells. Normally they do not trigger an immune response except in the case of auto-immune disease. **Non-self antigens** are part of the outer surfaces of viruses, bacteria, fungi and animal parasites, or may be toxins produced by pathogenic microorganisms. Their presence in the body normally provokes an immune response.

    Lymphocytes are types of white blood cells that recognise and react to antigens. They originate in the bone marrow from cells (**stem cells**)

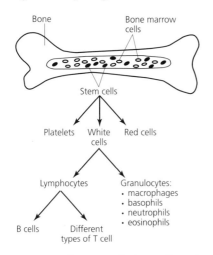

Figure 2.1 Development of white cells and other blood cells in the bone marrow.

Diseases where the patient makes antibodies which destroy his/her own tissues are called **auto-immune** diseases. For example, the disease **pernicious anaemia** is caused by the destruction of cells from the lining of the stomach which secrete a substance called **intrinsic factor** needed for the absorption of vitamin B_{12}. The victim's antibodies combine with intrinsic factor, preventing the uptake of vitamin B_{12}.

Pernicious anaemia is treated with injections of vitamin B_{12}. Patients improve rapidly, often reporting a marked feeling of well-being within 48 hours of treatment beginning. Treatment is given every few months for the rest of the patient's life.

that also make other blood cells (figure 2.1). However, unlike the other cells, lymphocytes migrate to the **spleen** and **lymph nodes** (figure 2.2) where they mature, and they are produced in large numbers throughout a person's life. Some lymphocytes pass through the **thymus** (shown in figure 2.2) on their way to the spleen and lymph nodes. They are called **T lymphocytes** or **T cells**. Processing in the thymus sensitises them so that they recognise specific antigens. Lymphocytes that migrate directly to the spleen and lymph nodes without passing through the thymus are called **B lymphocytes** or **B cells**.

Lymph bathes the body's cells in a solution of oxygen and nutrients. It drains from all of the body's tissues into the lymphatic system. This means that antigens from anywhere in the body are eventually detected

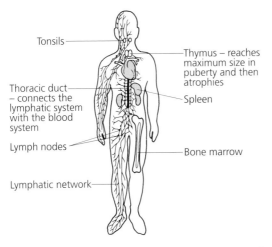

Figure 2.2 The lymphatic system. Lymphocytes are produced in the bone marrow and migrate to the lymph nodes, spleen and other lymphatic tissue throughout the body. (Lymphatic network shown on right-hand side of body only.) A lymph node is shown in more detail in figure 2.3.

by the T and B lymphocytes lodged in the lymph nodes. Figure 2.3 shows
how the cells respond.

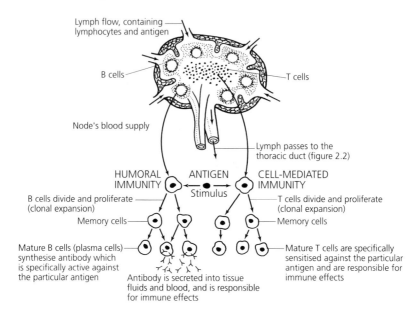

Figure 2.3 Section through a lymph node showing distribution of B cells and T
cells. The cells circulate in the blood and lymph. Lymph containing antigens
flows into the node. Following stimulation by contact with antigen, the B cells
and T cells respond by attacking the antigen, resulting in two categories of
immunity – humoral and cell-mediated.

Antibodies are a type of protein called **immunoglobulin**
(abbreviated to **Ig**), and form the gamma–globulin component of
plasma proteins. The main categories of immunoglobulin are:

IgG – represents many different antibodies and makes up 85% of
total immunoglobulin in circulation. Anti-rhesus factor (page
33) is an example of IgG.

IgM – made up of five IgG-type antibodies joined together. Anti-A
and anti-B (page 32) are examples.

IgE – involved in allergic responses, e.g. hay fever and asthma
(page 76).

IgD – function uncertain.

Humoral immunity

When a quantity of antigen (for example, on the cell surfaces of invading
bacteria) enters the lymph nodes, it combines with antigen-specific
receptors on the surfaces of the B lymphocytes. This activates the B

lymphocytes and, as a result, they divide and enlarge to become **plasma cells** which produce the **antibody** specific to the antigen that triggered the response. The antibodies circulate in the blood.

Cell-mediated immunity

Unlike B lymphocytes, T lymphocytes do not secrete antibodies. However, like B lymphocytes, each type has surface receptors that bind to a particular antigen which may appear, for example, on the surfaces of virally infected cells.

Binding to the antigen activates the T lymphocytes, which divide forming populations of cells with different functions. For example, some T lymphocytes (called **T-helper** cells) control the production of antibodies by B lymphocytes; others (called **T-cytotoxic** cells) directly destroy virally infected cells. Sometimes the actions of T lymphocytes affect a person adversely. For example, they are involved in auto-immune diseases (page 22), **rejection** of organ transplants (page 29) and **hypersensitivity** reactions.

2.2 Destruction of antigens

When the body is challenged with non-self antigens, the immune response swings into action (figure 2.4). Notice that the antibodies produced by the

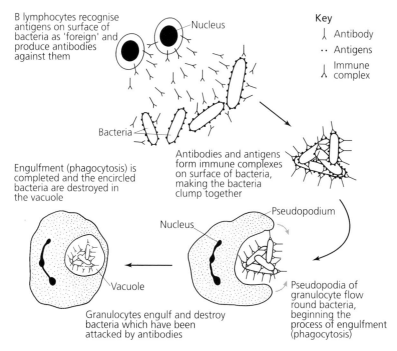

B lymphocytes recognise antigens on surface of bacteria as 'foreign' and produce antibodies against them

Nucleus

Key

ʎ Antibody

·· Antigens

ʎ Immune complex

Bacteria

Antibodies and antigens form immune complexes on surface of bacteria, making the bacteria clump together

Engulfment (phagocytosis) is completed and the encircled bacteria are destroyed in the vacuole

Nucleus

Pseudopodium

Vacuole

Granulocytes engulf and destroy bacteria which have been attacked by antibodies

Pseudopodia of granulocyte flow round bacteria, beginning the process of engulfment (phagocytosis)

Figure 2.4 Lymphocytes and granulocytes at work.

B lymphocytes stick to the antigens covering the surfaces of the invading bacteria, and form combinations called **immune complexes** which make the bacteria clump together. Notice also that the lymphocytes work with **granulocytes**: another category of white blood cell produced in the bone marrow (figure 2.1). Together, lymphocytes and granulocytes work quickly to destroy the 'foreign' material.

In reality, however, events are much more complex than this. Bear in mind the summary (figure 2.4) as you look at figure 2.5, which shows the different reactions of the immune response. Consider first the various types of granulocyte (figure 2.1). The activity of a type called **basophils** is mediated by the immunoglobulin IgE (page 24). Antigens binding to IgE, which coats the basophils, stimulate the basophils to release different substances, e.g. **histamine**. Histamine promotes the movement of blood plasma containing white blood cells into infected tissues. The movement provokes an **inflammatory** reaction with swelling, redness and heat at the site of infection. This is the basis of allergic responses such as hay fever and **asthma** (page 76). Blood plasma also contains at least 15 different proteins called **complement**. The process by which non-self antigens are coated with complement and antibodies is called **opsonisation**. Opsonisation helps other types of granulocyte called **neutrophils** and **macrophages** target invading pathogens. It also stimulates the formation of pseudopodia and therefore promotes **phagocytosis** (figure 2.4).

Figure 2.5 shows that the various types of lymphocyte and

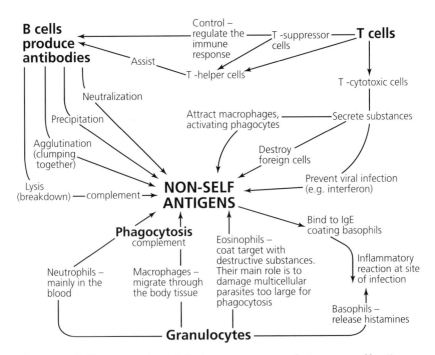

Figure 2.5 Different reactions of the immune response destroy non-self antigens.

granulocyte have different functions which work together to ensure the body's survival in the face of attack by pathogens. This is one reason why most of us remain healthy most of the time. Sometimes pathogens may take hold temporarily and we are ill. Normally, however, the immune system soon gains the upper hand and we quickly recover, though sometimes with the help of drugs. Occasionally the effects of pathogens are **chronic** (long term) and, when the immune system is damaged (e.g. by HIV), may be fatal.

2.3 Immunological memory

On first encounter, it may take the body a few days to produce antibodies against an infection. This is known as the **primary** immune response. However, the next encounter with the same organism results in a much quicker response. This **secondary** immune response provides evidence for **immunological memory**. B lymphocyte and T lymphocyte **memory** cells left over from the earlier division of lymphocytes (called **clonal expansion**) are activated. They divide quickly (second clonal expansion) on re-exposure to the same antigen. Figure 2.6 summarises the sequence of events.

Memory cells are specific to particular antigens and it is due to their action that we do not usually catch mumps or chicken-pox more than once in a lifetime. The rapid response of immunological memory destroys the viruses before they make us ill. Having the disease, therefore, and recovering from it makes a person **resistant** to the infection. This is the basis of **active immunity.**

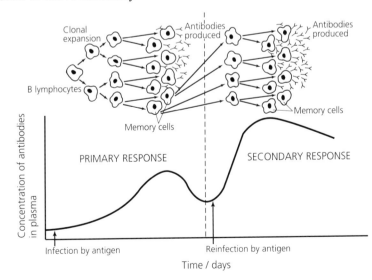

Figure 2.6 Primary and secondary immune responses.

Most of the cells produced during the **primary** immune response die after a few weeks. The persistence of memory cells means that it is not necessary for there to be large numbers of each specific lymphocyte in circulation all the time. The **secondary** response means that defences against a particular reinvader can be called upon quickly.

2.4 What makes antibodies specific?

Figure 2.7 shows the structure of an antibody molecule. Each molecule consists of polypeptide chains – two identical **heavy** chains and two identical **light** chains joined in a Y shape. The two arms, which combine with antigens, have the same structure. Comparing the amino acid sequences of the arms of many different antibody molecules shows that the sequences vary from one type of antibody to another. The arms, therefore, are called the **variable (V)** regions and are the basis of antibody specificity. Variability permits a flexible response by the body to the arrival of antigens. A particular antigen stimulates the production of the antibody whose shape fits that antigen and no other. An antibody and antigen will only combine to form an **immune complex** if their shape and structure match. This is why, for example, antibodies produced against typhoid bacteria will not attack pneumonia bacteria. Each of us is capable of producing tens of millions of different types of antibodies to challenge all the antigens we are ever likely to meet.

The stem of the antibody molecule does not combine with the antigen. It varies much less between different antibodies and is, therefore, called the **constant (C)** region of the molecule.

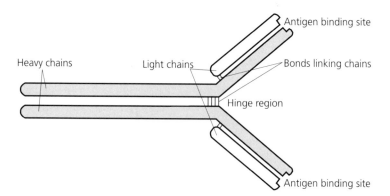

Figure 2.7 Basic antibody structure. The flexible hinge region enables both binding sites to make contact with the matching area of the antigen being attacked.

2.5 Transplant rejection

Antigens are not only found on bacteria and viruses: mammalian cell membranes also contain antigens called **histocompatibility** antigens. These proteins are the products of the genes of the **major histocompatibility complex (MHC)**. In humans, the MHC is the **human lymphocyte antigens (HLA)** gene cluster on chromosome 6 (page 126). The HLA system contains an enormous variety of antigens, and even closely related people (with the exception of identical twins) rarely have identical HLA types.

Because the HLA system regulates T lymphocyte activity and because it varies so much between individuals, it is not surprising that HLA antigens in transplanted organs activate an immune response in the recipient. The recipient's lymphocytes attack the transplanted organ and cause tissue rejection. The HLA molecules in the donor's organs are called **transplantation antigens**.

Preventing rejection

There are different ways of reducing the chance of rejection:
- **Tissue typing** identifies the different histocompatibility antigens in the donor and the recipient. Transplantation is carried out only if the proteins are very similar or identical. In this way humoral immunity responses and cell-mediated immunity responses (see figure 2.3) are minimised. Some HLA antigens produce stronger rejection reactions than others. Matching these antigens between donor and recipient is therefore especially important if the transplant is to stand a chance of long-term success.
- **Immunosuppressive drugs** inhibit the recipient's immune system and therefore prevent an immune response even if the histocompatibility antigens in the donor tissues are different from the histocompatibility antigens in the recipient. These drugs act primarily against dividing cells – not only lymphocytes but any types of body cell. The damage these drugs may cause to other dividing tissues (e.g. the lining of the gut) therefore limits their use.
- **Cyclosporine**, extracted from the fungus *Trichoderma polysporum*, was developed originally as an anti-fungal agent. The drug is more active against lymphocytes than against other cells and is, therefore, generally less poisonous than other immuno-suppressive drugs to other tissues of the body. When administered at the time of transplantation, it prevents the recipient's T lymphocytes from becoming active against the antigens in the transplanted tissue.

  Because cyclosporine and other immunosuppressive drugs

reduce the effectiveness of the immune system, the recipient is more susceptible to infections. If infection occurs, then use of the drugs may have to be suspended, but this increases the likelihood of immune reactions developing, leading to rejection of the transplant.

2.6 Immunisation

The development of active immunity to disease-causing microorganisms is possible through **immunisation**. A vaccine is the substance injected or swallowed which causes the development of active immunity, and immunisation (vaccination) is the process of being immunised.

Most vaccines are made by one of the following methods:

- *Dead microorganisms* killed by heat or the addition of chemicals such as formaldehyde. The dead microorganisms do not cause disease, but the structures of the microorganisms' surface molecules are preserved and can therefore act as antigens to stimulate antibody production in the recipient. Examples include the whooping cough vaccine and the Salk vaccine against poliomyelitis.
- *A weakened live form of a microorganism.* Vaccines made like this are called **attenuated** vaccines. The attenuated microorganism infects the recipient, stimulating the production of antibodies, but does not cause disease. Examples are the BCG vaccine against tuberculosis and the Sabin vaccine taken orally against poliomyelitis.
- *Substances made from parts of the microorganism or its toxins.* Inactivation makes the substances (called **toxoids**) harmless, but does not affect their role as antigens stimulating the production of antibodies in the recipient. Examples include the tetanus and diphtheria vaccines.

The advantages of live attenuated vaccines are that:

- attenuated microorganisms multiply in the recipient so that only a low dose of vaccine is needed to deliver sufficient antigen for an effective immune reaction to occur;
- live multiplying microorganisms produce long-term protection, probably because they stimulate the production of memory cells.

However, there are disadvantages:

- mutation of the attenuated microorganism may make the vaccine ineffective or, very occasionally, the microorganism may revert to the disease-causing form;
- live vaccines must be stored in cool conditions.

Whether killed or live microorganisms are used, vaccines often contain fragments of the cells in which the viruses or bacteria have been cultured. These impurities may cause unwanted or even dangerous side effects. New types of vaccine, based on a particular protein or on a small component of the infective microorganism, are being developed. Called **subunit vaccines**, they are designed to stimulate the production of antibodies in the recipient, yet avoid the unwanted or dangerous side effects of whole vaccines.

Even though vaccines made by the methods just described protect millions of people worldwide from serious disease, minute risks remain. For example, microorganisms used to make vaccines may survive the production process, and they may infect people working in production who, despite strict safety precautions, may come into contact with them. **Genetic engineering** is helping to reduce even these minute risks (page 131).

What effect does a vaccine have? Once given, the antigens in the vaccine stimulate the recipient's lymphocytes to produce antibodies. When, at some later date, the same active, harmful microorganisms invade the body, the antibodies made in response to the vaccine swing into action and destroy the microorganisms.

The active immunity produced by vaccines can protect a person from disease for a long time, although several more vaccinations called **boosters** may be needed after the first one. Boosters keep up the level of antibodies and maintain a person's immunity.

Passive immunity

Not all vaccines contain antigens which stimulate the body's lymphocytes to produce antibodies. Instead, antibodies ready-made by other animals may be used to make vaccines. For example, anti-tetanus antibodies produced by horses may be included in anti-tetanus vaccines. The only problem with this is that people who suffer from asthma, or any other allergies, may react badly to the horse serum in which the anti-toxin is contained.

The bacterium which causes tetanus lives in the soil. It multiplies very rapidly where there is little air, such as in a deep wound. It acts so quickly that the body's lymphocytes do not have time to make antibodies against the bacterium's lethal toxin. This is why a patient with a deep, dirty cut that may be contaminated with soil is injected with a vaccine containing anti-tetanus antibodies which act immediately to stop the disease from developing. This type of immunity, which comes from antibodies made in another animal, is called **passive immunity.**

Unfortunately, passive immunity does not last long because the body recognises that the horse anti-tetanus antibodies are non-self antigens and destroys them. However, the immunity lasts long enough to give immediate protection to patients at risk from infection with tetanus bacteria. A tetanus vaccine is now available which is made from attenuated tetanus bacteria. This gives longer-lasting active immunity because the lymphocytes 'learn' to make their own antibodies.

Passive immunity is important for newborn mammals. When suckled they receive antibodies from their mother's milk which protect them from disease-causing microorganisms when they are very young. By the time this protection wears off, the offspring are older and able to make their own antibodies. Before birth, mammals also receive antibodies across the placenta from their mother's bloodstream.

2.7 Blood groups

Although red blood cells all look alike under the microscope, they carry different antigens (called **agglutinogens**) on the cell surface. Certain antibodies (called **agglutinins**) may also be present in the plasma. People can be placed into one of a number of **blood groups**, depending on the presence or absence of particular antigens and antibodies. Table 2.1 gives some examples.

The most important blood group systems are the ABO and rhesus systems. In the ABO system people carry one, both or neither of two antigens called **A** and **B**. Their plasma contains one, both or neither of two antibodies called **anti-A** and **anti-B**. These antibodies appear soon after birth and are called **alloantibodies** as distinct from immune antibodies which are produced as a result of the immune response.

People whose red cells carry antigen A belong to blood group A, those with antigen B belong to group B and those with both antigens belong to group AB. People that have red cells with neither antigen belong to group O. The distribution of anti-A and anti-B antibodies is such that

Table 2.1. The red cell antigens of some of the blood group systems found in humans

Blood group system	Most important antigens present
ABO	A_1, A_2, B, etc.
Rhesus	D, C, E c, e, etc.
Kell	Kk, Kp^2, Kp^b, Js^a, Js^b
Duffy	Fy^2, Fy^b
Kidd	Jk^a, Jk^b

they do not normally come into contact with their specific antigen. The different combinations of antigens and antibodies are summarised in table 2.2.

The A, B and O blood groups were first described in 1900. Soon after their discovery, it was noticed that when mixed with anti-A antibodies, group A red cells from some people reacted more strongly than group A red cells from others. In 1911 these observations led to the discovery of A and AB subgroups (table 2.3).

The rhesus antigen

The red blood cells of some people carry another antigen known as the **rhesus D antigen**, so-called because it was first discovered in 1940 in the blood of rhesus monkeys. People with rhesus D antigen on their red cells are rhesus D positive (**RhD+**); those without are rhesus D negative (**RhD−**). Because the rhesus D antigen is distributed on red cells independently of the ABO antigens, individuals of any ABO blood group can be either RhD+ or RhD−.

People do not make spontaneous antibodies to the rhesus D antigen. However, RhD+ blood given to a RhD− patient stimulates the B lymphocytes in the recipient to make antibodies against the rhesus D antigen. Although not harmful during the first transfusion, the antibodies

Table 2.2. Blood groups

Antigen on red blood cells	Antibody in plasma	Blood group	% of UK Caucasian population
A	anti-B	A	46
B	anti-A	B	8
A and B	none	AB	2
neither A nor B	anti-A and anti-B	O	44

Table 2.3. ABO subgroups

Group	Subgroup	% of UK total population
A	A_1	33.5
	A_2	8.5
AB	A_1B	2.7
	A_2B	0.3

remain in the blood and will react against any subsequent transfusions of RhD+ blood. This reaction is less severe than in a mismatch between ABO blood groups, but should be avoided in people who are already unwell. it is also important to avoid RhD mismatching when transfusing female patients of childbearing age. RhD– mismatching is a major risk during the second pregnancy of a RhD– woman carrying a RhD+ baby. A dominant allele (page 117) codes for the rhesus D antigen, and providing the parental rhesus groups are known, it is possible to predict the rhesus group of the child.

Usually the RhD+ fetus does not affect the blood of the RhD– mother because their blood systems are separate. However, occasionally small amounts of blood leak from the fetus into the mother's blood through the placenta causing the mother to produce rhesus D antibodies. These antibodies may cross the placenta and destroy the red cells of the fetus. In the first pregnancy, the fetus is usually unaffected. However, in successive pregnancies antibodies accumulated by the mother may destroy so many red cells in the fetus that it dies in the uterus or is born anaemic and jaundiced (jaundiced babies are yellow because of the substances released by the destroyed red cells). The condition is known as **haemolytic disease of the newborn**. Babies affected by this receive transfusions at birth to replace the affected blood.

Haemolytic disease of the newborn used to be a major cause of death among newborn babies. However, there is now a solution to the problem. When a RhD– mother gives birth to her first RhD+ baby, she is injected with antiserum containing anti-D antibodies within three days of birth. These antibodies destroy any RhD+ that may have leaked from the fetus into her blood during pregnancy, before the RhD+ red cells have time to stimulate the mother's immune system. During the course of the next few weeks, the injected antibodies are broken down so that none remain to affect the next pregnancy.

T H R E E

The control of bleeding

A cut is the signal that begins a series of events which eventually stops the bleeding:

- **constriction** of the ends of the damaged blood vessels reduces the loss of blood;
- **clotting** – blood leaking from damaged blood vessels solidifies and forms a clot which plugs the wound, sealing it against infection from pathogens.

3.1 Blood clotting

The release of certain substances into the blood plasma begins the process of clotting. **Serotonin** (5-hydroxytryptamine) causes constriction of the damaged blood vessels. Other substances react with blood factors in the plasma, beginning a cascade of at least 15 chemical reactions that ends with the soluble plasma protein **fibrinogen** changing into insoluble **fibrin**. Figure 3.1 shows the process of clot formation. Production of the lipoprotein **thromboplastin** is a key stage in the process. It requires various substances including **factor VIII** in the plasma. Thromboplastin originates from:

- *damaged tissues* outside the blood vessels (the **extrinsic mechanism**);
- *platelets* in the blood (the **intrinsic mechanism**).

Whether thromboplastin is extrinsic or intrinsic in origin, different blood clotting factors including calcium ions (Ca^{2+} – **factor IV**) are required for it to convert the inactive blood protein **prothrombin** from the liver into its active form **thrombin**. Thrombin acts on fibrinogen (also produced in the liver), converting it to insoluble fibrin. The fibrin forms a mesh of fibres across the wound and traps **red cells** and platelets, forming a plug-like clot. The plug prevents further loss of blood from the blood vessels while repair of the injury takes place.

Healing starts when bleeding stops. The healing process is complex. It includes dissolution (dissolving) of the clot by an enzyme called **fibrinolysin** released from white blood cells: a process called **fibrinolysis**.

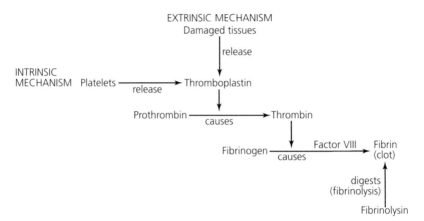

Figure 3.1 Summary of reactions that cause the formation of a blood clot.

First aid to control bleeding

Blood loss from a deep cut may be too great for a clot to form without help. First aid aims to control bleeding and so help clotting take place:

- *pressure* on the wound reduces blood loss and gives time for the blood to clot;
- *elevation* of a cut arm or leg reduces bleeding by lowering blood pressure in the joints;
- *dressing* with a sterile medicated dressing stops the bleeding.

Most cuts and scratches are not serious and clotting soon stops any bleeding. First aid aims to clean and dress the wound as quickly as possible to reduce the risk of infection.

3.2 Anticoagulants

A clot inside a blood vessel is called a **thrombus** (chapter 4). **Anticoagulant** drugs help prevent clots from forming in blood vessels (table 3.1).

Patients are often treated with a combination of **heparin** and **warfarin**. Heparin has a very short biological half-life (two hours), and since prothrombin is produced continuously in the liver, the effect of heparin is short lived. The effect of warfarin is longer lasting because it affects vitamin K synthesis which is essential for the action of some coagulation factors.

The survival of heart attack victims is improved by treating them with drugs that break down blood clots in the coronary arteries. The most widely used drug is **streptokinase** which is given in a saline drip as soon

Table 3.1. Anticoagulants in common use

Anticoagulant	Effect
Therapeutic	
Warfarin	Prevents production of prothrombin by the liver
Heparin	Counteracts thrombin
In vitro *use only*	
EDTA (ethylene-diamenetetracetic acid)	Lowers the concentration of calcium ions in the plasma
Sodium citrate	Binds calcium ions, reducing concentration in plasma

as possible after the onset of symptoms. Streptokinase promotes fibrinolysis (figure 3.1). Giving aspirin in combination with streptokinase can further improve the chances of survival. Aspirin inhibits platelet **agglutination** (sticking together) and therefore helps prevent clots from forming.

3.3 Haemophilia

Some people suffer from a disease that causes them to bleed copiously if they injure themselves because their blood does not clot properly. This disease is called **haemophilia**, and sufferers may lose a lot of blood from even a small cut. Haemophilia is a genetic disease that is sex-linked (chapter 11). The allele responsible is recessive and located on the X chromosome, so it is almost always males that are affected.

Clotting time for a haemophiliac may be up to 12 hours compared with 5–10 minutes for a healthy person. Internal bleeding into the joints can also be a major problem, starting as soon as a child suffering from haemophilia begins to walk. Haemophilia A is the most common form of the disease. It results from the absence of factor VIII, needed to change fibrinogen into fibrin (figure 3.1), from the blood. Haemophiliacs with the A form of the disease are treated with injections of factor VIII from blood donated through the Blood Transfusion Service. Genetically engineered factor VIII (chapter 12) can be expressed in the milk of sheep produced from fertilised eggs into which copies of the clotting factor gene have been injected. Factor VIII produced in this way is being evaluated for use in treatment. The sheep are **transgenic** – so-called because a 'foreign' human gene (**transgene**) has been introduced and integrated into the sheep's genotype (page 132). The clotting factor transgene is present in their sex cells and can be inherited by future generations.

Although only low levels of factor VIII have been produced by this method so far, transgenic sheep and other transgenic animals promise to be an important means by which human healthcare products are produced in the future. In the case of factor VIII, an important potential advantage is the prevention of disease transmission via blood products.

Factor IX is absent from the blood in cases of haemophilia B. The symptoms are the same as for haemophilia A, and both forms of the disease are managed in a similar way. Injections of factor IX concentrate (or infusions of plasma containing factor IX) are used to control bleeding.

F O U R

Heart disease

4.1 What is heart disease?

The walls of the heart are very thick. Food and oxygen dissolved in the blood cannot pass quickly enough from inside the heart to all of the heart muscles by diffusion alone. The **coronary arteries** running over the surface of the heart transport blood, carrying dissolved food and oxygen, to the heart muscles.

The smooth inner wall of healthy blood vessels allows blood to flow easily through them. Anticoagulants such as **heparin** (from the liver) and **prostacyclin** (from the lining of blood vessels) prevent blood from clotting inside vessels. However, deposits of a fatty material called **plaque** can roughen the inner wall. As plaque builds up it causes a type of 'hardening' of the arteries called **arteriosclerosis**. The roughened blood vessels become narrower, blood flows through the vessels more slowly and the release of prostacyclin is inhibited. As a result:

- platelets (page 35) clump together (**agglutinate**);
- **thromboplastin** is released – the enzyme that begins the process of blood clotting.

These events increase the risk of blood clotting and blocking blood vessels. If an artery is blocked completely, then food and oxygen cannot reach the tissue that the artery supplies. The tissue is damaged and may die (**infarction**). The clot is called a **thrombus** and the blockage a **thrombosis.**

Sometimes a thrombus may be dislodged and carried in the bloodstream. The mobile thrombus is called an **embolus**. If an embolus then lodges in a blood vessel, it may cause a blockage called an **embolism**.

Arteriosclerosis in the coronary arteries is one cause of heart disease. If the diameter of the arteries is reduced by 50% or more then breathlessness and a cramp-like pain may be brought on by quick walking, anger, excitement or anything else that makes the heart work harder than usual. The pain is called **angina** and is the heart's response to being starved of the oxygen that blood carries. Angina usually goes away after a few minutes rest. People live with some types of angina for years, but other types get worse and may later result in a heart attack (**coronary thrombosis or myocardial infarction**).

Treating angina

Different types of **nitrate drug** have been used for many years to treat the symptoms of angina. They relieve chest pain and, if taken beforehand, allow people with angina to take moderate exercise. **Glycerol trinitrate** is one of the most effective nitrate drugs. It dilates (makes wider) the coronary arteries, improving the blood supply to the heart muscles and reducing the work of the left ventricle.

When a coronary artery (or arteries) becomes blocked, a heart attack occurs. The blood supply to the heart is interrupted and pain usually grips the victim's chest, spreading to the arms, neck and jaw. Other signs of heart attack are:

- feeling sick and faint;
- sweating;
- breathlessness;
- a weak, irregular, fast pulse;
- a pale skin, and lips and fingertips tinged blue (**cyanosis**). This is due to blood not reaching the body's surface.

Sometimes a heart attack is so severe that **cardiac arrest** occurs. The victim's heart stops beating altogether. The person becomes unconscious, the pulse and breathing stop and cyanosis is severe. In such cases, it is essential to get the heart beating again within a few minutes, otherwise the person will die.

FIRST AID AND THE HEART ATTACK VICTIM
If you think a person has had a heart attack, call urgently for a doctor or ambulance. Comfort the victim until medical help arrives. The flow chart will help you decide what more to do. Remember – only undertake first aid if it is really necessary to do so.

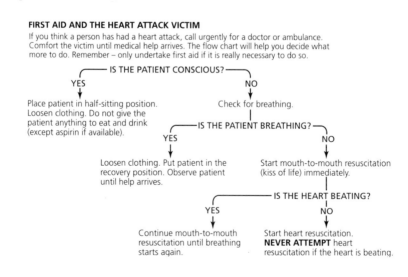

IS THE PATIENT CONSCIOUS?

YES → Place patient in half-sitting position. Loosen clothing. Do not give the patient anything to eat and drink (except aspirin if available).

NO → Check for breathing.

IS THE PATIENT BREATHING?

YES → Loosen clothing. Put patient in the recovery position. Observe patient until help arrives.

NO → Start mouth-to-mouth resuscitation (kiss of life) immediately.

IS THE HEART BEATING?

YES → Continue mouth-to-mouth resuscitation until breathing starts again.

NO → Start heart resuscitation. **NEVER ATTEMPT** heart resuscitation if the heart is beating.

4.2 Deaths from heart disease

In the UK, disease of the heart and blood vessels accounts for about a quarter of all deaths, and is the largest single cause of death and the main cause of early death. Figure 4.1 shows a similar pattern of mortality in other developed countries of the world. The problem is not new, but has greatly increased in scale since the beginning of the twentieth century.

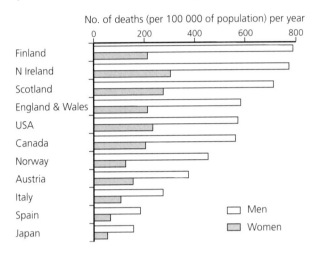

Figure 4.1 Deaths from heart disease (35–74 year olds) for developed countries. (Based on figures from the World Health Organisation.)

In many less developed countries heart disease is quite rare. Two questions arise:

- Why do people living in prosperous, industrialised countries (although Japan is an exception) seem more likely to develop heart disease?
- Why has the risk increased over the past hundred years?

Risk factors

Some of the causes of heart disease have been identified by comparing populations with high rates of heart disease with populations that have low rates. When a difference between groups is found that might explain why some people are more likely to develop heart disease than others, it is called a **risk factor**.

Three risk factors are unavoidable: our sex, age and the genes we inherit. Figure 4.2 summarises the evidence. People in these categories do not necessarily die from heart disease – the risk factors are controllable, and people who live sensibly can increase their chances of reaching a ripe old age. Living sensibly means reducing our exposure to the controllable risk factors in our daily lives.

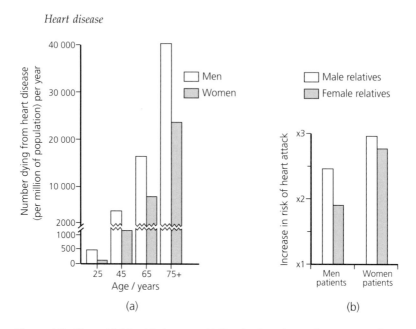

Figure 4.2 Unavoidable risk factors: (*a*) Deaths from heart disease according to age and sex, for England and Wales; (*b*) Relatives of people who have a heart attack are more likely to suffer one themselves. Notice that the relatives of women patients are more at risk than the relatives of men patients. Is the inheritance of a tendency to have heart attacks sex-linked (chapter 11)?

4.3 Links between diet and heart disease

People who eat too much fat and sugar tend to put on weight. Excessively overweight (**obese**) people have a higher risk of heart disease.

Many people are conscious of their weight. Terms like 'saturated fats', 'polyunsaturated fats', 'cholesterol levels', 'fish oil' and 'sunflower oil' become a familiar part of a person's vocabulary when weight watching. Advertisements and nutrition experts bombard us with advice about dietary fats, and the relation between fat intake and heart disease. We need some fat in our diet for good health, so what are the facts?

Cholesterol levels

Cholesterol is a clear, oily liquid and is often quoted as an important culprit linked with heart disease. It is a part of animal cell membranes and a component of steroid hormones such as **testosterone** and **oestrogen.**

Large amounts of cholesterol are found in plaque deposits blocking blood vessels, and the more cholesterol there is in the blood, the greater the risk of heart disease (figure 4.3). Eating foods containing a lot of **saturated** fat seems to be the problem. Saturated fats can raise the natural level of cholesterol in the blood.

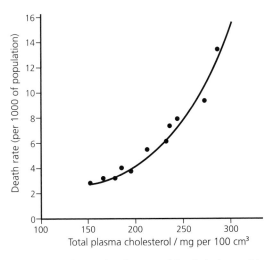

Figure 4.3 The relationship between blood cholesterol levels and risk of death from coronary heart disease.

However, the story is not so straightforward as may seem at first sight. Cholesterol is synthesised by the liver from fragments of saturated fatty acids. The liver makes less cholesterol as the intake of saturated fat and cholesterol increases. These adjustments by the liver help keep blood cholesterol levels within normal range. If our intake of saturated fat and cholesterol is more than the liver can adjust for, then high blood cholesterol levels may result.

Even so, not everyone with a high fat/cholesterol diet will develop high blood cholesterol levels. The reasons are not known for certain, but it seems that some people can break down cholesterol more effectively than others. Also, in some people, the liver produces less cholesterol.

High blood cholesterol levels, therefore, need not have a dietary link. Cholesterol levels can be increased by:

- genetic characteristics which cause the liver to produce too much cholesterol;
- oral contraceptive pills;
- drugs used to treat high blood pressure.

Even if people with a genetic tendency to make too much cholesterol stick to a low-cholesterol diet, they still generally have blood cholesterol levels higher than most other people.

Role of lipoproteins

Cholesterol is insoluble and transported in the blood bound to a protein **carrier**. The cholesterol/protein combination forms a **lipoprotein**. There are four main types of lipoprotein, each one consisting of varying amounts of protein, triglyceride and cholesterol. They are identified by density – their weight relative to the weight of other substances of equal volume. Two of them – **low-density lipoproteins (LDL)** and **high-density lipoproteins (HDL)** – are especially important in the development of heart disease:

- *Low-density lipoproteins* contain the highest proportion of cholesterol of all the lipoproteins. They transport most of the cholesterol in the blood and increase the rate of build-up of plaque. Raised cholesterol levels are almost always associated with raised LDL levels, and indicate increased risk of heart attack.
- *High-density lipoproteins* contain the most protein. They lower the risk of heart disease by removing cholesterol from the blood, slowing down plaque formation. The cholesterol is transported to the liver where it is broken down and excreted.

Assessing the risk

Measuring the relative proportions of LDL and HDL in the blood is a better risk indicator for heart disease than measuring cholesterol levels alone. For example, a person with a low total blood cholesterol level but a high proportion of LDL may be more at risk than somebody with high total blood cholesterol but a high proportion of HDL. Different studies show that HDL levels are a reliable indicator of the risk of heart disease: high levels of HDL reduce risk, low levels of HDL increase risk. Women generally have higher levels of HDL than men, which perhaps accounts for why they suffer from less heart disease. Exercise (chapter 5) and modest amounts of alcohol also raise HDL with similar benefits.

Reducing risk

Although more research is needed to sort out the uncertainties of dietary risk assessment, there is some evidence that the risk of heart disease decreases with reduced blood cholesterol levels. This can be achieved by:

- *Changing the diet* – reducing the intake of saturated fat is an important positive step to take. Eating fish and bran from whole oats (unrefined porridge, oat biscuits, etc.) is also beneficial. Different types of fish (especially mackerel, trout, herring and tuna) are a rich source of **omega-3 fatty acids**. Research indicates that if 4 grams of omega-3 fatty acids are eaten with food each day (equivalent to about two fish meals a week), then the build up of plaque and blood pressure (page 46) is reduced. This may explain why Innuits (Eskimos), who traditionally eat a lot of fish, are at low risk of developing heart disease. Oat bran binds with cholesterol, partly blocking its absorption through

the intestinal wall. As little as two tablespoons of oat bran a day have been found to reduce blood cholesterol levels significantly.
- *Drugs* that reduce cholesterol levels – these have side effects (such as increasing blood pressure) that make their use worthwhile only if changes in diet have no effect. They are also expensive.

What is the most effective action for reducing blood cholesterol levels and therefore the risk of heart disease? Research suggests that total food energy intake should consist of no more than 30% as fat, and the fat that is eaten should contain slightly more unsaturated fat than saturated fat. Monounsaturated fats lower blood cholesterol levels, but less so than polyunsaturated fats.

4.4 Links between smoking and heart disease

Smoking is one of the greatest causes of preventable death worldwide. Each year in Britain about 110 000 people die early because they smoke cigarettes. Nearly 50% of these early deaths are from diseases of the heart and blood vessels.

A lit cigarette gives out over a thousand chemicals, many of which are extremely harmful. **Nicotine** and **carbon monoxide,** in particular, affect the heart and blood vessels.
- *Nicotine* is one of the most powerful poisons known. It raises pulse rate and blood pressure, making people whose blood pressure is already high (page 47) even more at risk from heart disease.
- *Carbon monoxide* is a gas that combines with haemoglobin in red blood cells, reducing the level of oxygen in the blood. This means that the heart must work harder to supply the tissues and organs of the body with the oxygen they need. Plaque may develop because of damage to the lining of the blood vessels.

Smokers of all ages are at greater risk of dying from heart disease than non-smokers of the same age (figure 4.4). Also, the more heavily you smoke the more likely you are to die young from heart disease.

The campaign against smoking has been fought hard for a long time. Between 1972 and 1982, cigarette smoking among men and women in Britain dropped by almost a third. The proportion of people who smoke cigarettes continues to decline in all social groups, although cigarette smoking is still common among schoolchildren. The UK government's target in the next few years is to reduce prevalence among 11 to 15 year olds by at least a third. The overall message is clear – do not start smoking. It is bad for your health, and no longer has a positive 'image'.

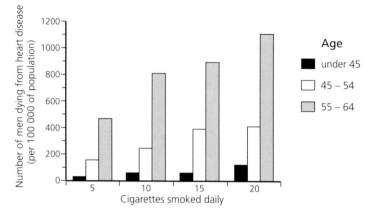

Figure 4.4 Smoking and the risk of death from heart disease among men.
Source: the Royal College of Physicians.

4.5 Links between blood pressure and heart disease

Blood pressure results from the heart pumping blood into the blood vessels against the resistance of the narrow vessels in particular. It can be measured with an instrument called a **sphygmomanometer** or with a digital device that fits over the finger. Two readings are taken:

- **systolic blood pressure** which is the pressure of blood when the heart contracts;
- **diastolic blood pressure** which is the pressure of blood when the heart relaxes.

The normal ranges of systolic and diastolic pressures depend on sex, age, health and general fitness. Anything that makes the heart beat faster (e.g. exercise and anger) will raise blood pressure, but readings will soon return to normal in a healthy person.

Risks of high blood pressure

Constant high blood pressure (**hypertension**) is harmful. It makes the heart work harder and causes the arteries to narrow because they 'fur up' with plaque more quickly. A vicious circle begins: so that enough blood reaches the body's tissues and organs, blood pressure increases further, resulting in more damage as plaque builds up more quickly. Eventually plaque may block the coronary arteries causing a heart attack, or the overworked heart may fail altogether. High blood pressure can also damage the kidneys and eyes, and increase the risk of rupture of an artery in the brain (**stroke** or **cerebral haemorrhage**).

Whether it is systolic pressure or diastolic pressure which is raised, the risk of heart disease is increased. For example, there is a 20% probability of death in middle age within five years if diastolic pressures above 110 mm of mercury remain untreated.

Causes of hypertension

Few young people have high blood pressure, but after the age of 35 it becomes more common. More than 25% of men and women aged 55 upwards are thought to suffer from hypertension. Research shows that life-style can have an important effect:

- *Obesity* – different studies show that losing 3 kg body weight typically reduces systolic blood pressure by 7 mm of mercury and diastolic blood pressure by 4 mm of mercury.
- *Salt* – a substantial reduction in salt intake reduces blood pressure, though it may make food unattractive at first. Moderate reduction of salt in the diet (e.g. by not adding salt to food and avoiding heavily salted 'convenience' foods) can be helpful.
- *Alcohol* – drinking the equivalent of four pints of beer daily (80 g alcohol per day) or more raises blood pressure, especially in people who are already hypertensive. Blood pressure falls within hours after a person stops drinking alcohol. There is some evidence which suggests that modest intake of alcohol helps protect against heart disease. However, hypertensive patients should try to reduce alcohol intake to no more than the equivalent of one daily pint of beer.
- *Smoking* – cigarette smokers, especially, are at risk from hypertension. Also, smokers respond less well to drugs designed to reduce hypertension.

Regular exercise and relaxation can also help to reduce blood pressure (page 52). If high blood pressure is treated, then the risk of heart disease is reduced and the outlook for the patient is much improved.

Treating hypertension

In people with mild hypertension, blood pressure can usually be controlled without using drugs. The changes in life-style outlined above often bring about the desired result. However, if hypertension persists, then different drugs (**antihypertensives**) are available and can be tailored to the patient's individual circumstances.

The underlying principle in the treatment of hypertension is **step care**: treatment begins with one drug, and other drugs are then added 'stepwise' until satisfactory control of blood pressure is achieved.

Beta (ß) blockers are antihypertensive drugs in common use. They work by **competitively inhibiting** the action of the **hormones** adrenaline and noradrenaline. These hormones bind with **adrenaline receptors**, which are protein molecules embedded in the surface cell membranes of heart muscle and smooth muscle lining blood vessels. The receptors mediate the effect (help the action) of the hormones on the target tissues. The hormones constrict (narrow) blood vessels and increase the rate and strength of heartbeat – responses which both increase blood pressure. Beta blockers inhibit the action of adrenaline and noradrenaline by binding with ß receptors. Some block $ß_1$ receptors (heart) and $ß_2$ receptors (blood vessels), whereas others block $ß_1$ receptors only and are therefore selective for the heart. Beta blockers are thought to lower blood pressure by reducing the output of blood from the heart and by affecting the neural control of heartbeat.

Measuring and regulating heartbeat

The beating of the heart is controlled by a group of cells in the right auricle (atrium). These cells form a **natural pacemaker** called the **sinoatrial node**. Waves of electrical impulses spread rapidly from the pacemaker causing the right and left auricles to contract. About 100 milliseconds after the pacemaker fires, impulses stimulate another area of nodal tissue called the **atrioventricular node**, spread through special muscle fibres called the **bundle of His** and reach the walls of the right and left ventricles. The ventricles contract almost simultaneously. The atrioventricular node imposes a short delay between contraction of the auricles and that of the ventricles, ensuring that the beat of the auricles is completed before the beat of the ventricles begins.

The electrical changes occurring as the heart contracts reach the surface of the body. Electrodes placed appropriately on the body surface and connected to a recording instrument can measure the current. The output in the form of a trace helps to assess the heart's ability to initiate and transmit impulses, and therefore to assess heart fitness. The trace is called an **electrocardiogram** (ECG).

Occasionally the natural pacemaker goes wrong or its electrical impulses are blocked at the atrioventricular node and so do not pass properly from the auricles to the ventricles. The auricles and ventricles begin to beat out of sequence, and the heart rate slows down, causing drowsiness and shortage of breath. The heart may even stop beating. A small electronic pacemaker, which sends out electrical signals that stimulate the heart, helps keep the heart beating at a proper rate. Fitting one is fairly straightforward and can be carried out with the patient under local anaesthetic.

Physiological effects of exercise

Middle-aged people console themselves with the notion that 'life begins at forty', but ageing actually begins in the mid-twenties. By 'ageing' is meant loss of fitness rather than advancing years. Different aspects of fitness peak at different times, and individuals vary. For example, figure 5.1 shows the peak and decline of average muscular strength in men and women as they grow older.

Exercise helps slow the ageing process so that death from heart disease, for example, is less likely. Slowing down ageing does not mean a person lives longer (although this may happen), but rather that good health is enjoyed for a much greater part of their life.

5.1 Heart fitness

When there is an imbalance between the oxygen requirements of the heart and the amount of blood, with its load of oxygen, supplied to it by the

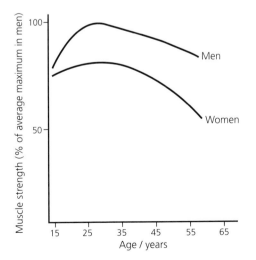

Figure 5.1 Relative muscle strength in men and women of different ages.

coronary arteries, the heart becomes starved of oxygen. The condition is called **ischaemia** and occurs in people with angina (page 39) or who exercise at levels which are unrealistically high with respect to their 'heart fitness'.

The **rate–pressure product** is an estimate of the heart's oxygen requirements. The higher the rate–pressure product, the higher the oxygen requirements of the heart. It is calculated as:

$$
\text{rate–pressure product} = \begin{matrix} \text{heart rate} \\ \text{(no. of beats per} \\ \text{minute – bpm)} \end{matrix} \times \begin{matrix} \text{Systolic blood} \\ \text{pressure (page 46)} \\ \text{(mm Hg)} \end{matrix}
$$

For example, someone exercising strenuously may typically have a heart rate of 190 bpm and systolic blood pressure of 220 mm Hg. Therefore:

$$
\text{rate–pressure product} = 190 \times 220 = 41\,800
$$

Reducing the heart rate or systolic blood pressure for a given workload will therefore reduce the oxygen requirements of the heart for that particular workload. This means that in situations where the blood supply to the heart may be limited (e.g. angina or during vigorous exercise), the threat to the heart of being deprived of oxygen is much less. For example, in the equation above, if the heart rate is reduced by 20 bpm to 170 bpm, then:

$$
\text{rate–pressure product} = 170 \times 220 = 37\,400
$$

a reduction in the oxygen requirement of the heart by more than 10%.

These examples show that for a given workload, reduction in the heart rate and/or systolic blood pressure makes an imbalance between the heart's supply of and demand for oxygen less likely. The health of the heart, therefore, is more certain.

Look at table 5.1. It shows how exercise may affect heart rate and therefore the rate–pressure product. Clearly the athlete's heart delivers blood, with its load of oxygen and dissolved food, to the body's tissues

Table 5.1. Oxygen requirements of the heart of a trained athlete compared with that of an untrained individual. (Assume a systolic blood pressure of 120 mm Hg in each case.)

	Heart rate (average)/bpm	*Rate–pressure product*
Trained athlete	38	4560
Untrained individual	72	8640

and organs more efficiently than the heart of a less active person. The athlete's **stroke volume** (volume of blood pumped from the heart with each beat) is greater, and so too, therefore, is **cardiac output** (volume of blood pumped from the heart each minute). At rest, an athlete's output may rise by 25%, increasing to 50% during vigorous exercise. These improvements are brought about by changes in the heart muscle. Regular exercise:

- increases heart size;
- improves the efficiency of the contraction of heart muscle;
- increases the volume of the chambers of the heart.

All these factors increase heart fitness. The combination of more efficient heart muscle and reduced oxygen demand by the heart at rest and during exercise makes life-threatening disturbances of the heart less likely.

5.2 Does exercise reduce the risk of heart disease?

Although exercise makes the heart more efficient, does it cut the risk of heart disease? The London Transport Study, published in 1953, was one of the first investigations into the relationship between physical activity and heart disease. The study looked at the occurrence of heart disease in 31 000 drivers and conductors over a two-year period. The conductors were more active than drivers, walking the length of the bus and up and down the stairs collecting passengers' fares. By comparison, drivers were sitting for most of the day. Analysis of the data showed that drivers had twice as many heart attacks, and twice as many fatal heart attacks, as conductors. In other words, conductors not only had fewer heart attacks than drivers, but what disease they did have was less likely to be fatal.

The London Transport Study pioneered research into the relationships between exercise and heart disease. The different studies that followed all suggest that regular exercise is an important protective measure that most of us can undertake.

Case study 1

Groups of monkeys were fed either on a diet rich in saturated fats or on a normal diet. The monkeys fed on the fat-rich diet were divided into a group that exercised regularly under controlled conditions, and a group that remained sedentary (unexercised). The monkeys fed on a normal diet were also sedentary – they acted as controls. Eighteen months later at post-mortem, there were striking differences between the monkeys on the fat-rich diet who exercised and those on the fat-rich diet who remained sedentary. The exercised monkeys had coronary arteries that were much wider and less 'furred up' with plaque than the sedentary monkeys, even though both groups had eaten food likely to increase plaque formation.

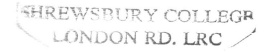
SHREWSBURY COLLEGE
LONDON RD. LRC

Case study 2

Other animal studies show that regular exercise may improve the supply of blood to the heart. After a heart attack, for example, exercise seems to encourage the growth of a new blood supply around blocked vessels. The new vessels eventually make up for the reduced blood supply through the diseased arteries.

The evidence from animal studies helps make the case for exercise: *regular exercise reduces the chance of heart disease developing, and helps restore the blood supply after a heart attack.*

5.3   Effects of exercise on blood pressure

Constantly raised blood pressure (page 46) is a major risk factor for heart disease. There is some evidence to suggest that regular exercise helps lower blood pressure in some people:

- blood pressure is lower in physically fit people compared with the unfit;
- if blood pressure is already raised, regular exercise can help to reduce it;
- exercise can help prevent high blood pressure from developing and thus reduce the risk of heart disease.

However, the observed effects may not be a direct result of the exercise itself, but may be partly due to loss of weight resulting from the exercise. Also, if blood pressure is already normal then exercise appears to have little effect.

5.4   Effects of exercise on blood fats

The importance of blood fats – especially cholesterol and lipoproteins – in the development of heart disease is discussed on pages 42–45. Generally, the more cholesterol there is in the blood, the more likely are blood vessels to 'fur up' with plaque deposits. High-density lipoproteins (HDL) slow down plaque formation.

Exercise has little direct effect on blood cholesterol. However, research has established a link between levels of HDL and exercise. For example, the HDL levels of medical students who exercised for 30 minutes 4 times a week for 7 weeks improved by 16%. Since the cholesterol in plaque seems to be removed by HDL and transported to the liver where it is broken down, it appears that exercise protects against the development of heart disease by raising HDL levels and thus reducing blood cholesterol.

5.5 Effects of exercise on blood clotting factors

Blood clots block blood vessels and may trigger a heart attack. Exercise reduces the tendency for blood to clot by increasing:

- *fibrinolysis* – the series of biochemical reactions that dissolve blood clots (page 35);
- *levels of prostacyclin* – secreted by the lining of blood vessels and preventing platelets from sticking together (page 39).

5.6 Effects of exercise on body weight

The media bombard us with body images. The message is: thin is beautiful. A bewildering array of slimming diets promise rapid weight loss for the millions of people trying to lose weight. Many make biological nonsense!

Water and glycogen account for most of the weight lost through 'crash dieting' and 95% of slimmers replace the weight in a short period of time (page 70). The only healthy way to lose weight is to make sure that energy intake (in food) is less than energy output (metabolism and physical activity). The options are:

- take more exercise, which increases energy output;
- eat less high-energy food, which decreases energy input;
- combine these two approaches.

If the intake of food energy is more than the energy used by the body, then the excess is stored as fatty adipose tissue. In other words, you become overweight and eventually obese.

Exercise reduces body fat by increasing **metabolic rate** (the rate at which a person uses energy). A high metabolic rate uses large amounts of energy and therefore helps control body fat. The effect persists – a raised metabolic rate continues for many hours after exercise has stopped. Regular exercise, therefore, can bring about a significant reduction in body weight. It can also lower blood pressure and raise levels of HDL. All of these effects mean that exercise helps reduce the risk of heart disease.

The body's energy needs

Metabolic rate, as a reflection of the body's energy needs, is at its lowest (**basal metabolic rate**) when a person is at rest or sleeping. Breathing, the repair and replacement of cells, heartbeat, growth and maintenance of body temperature are some of the activities that contribute to the basal metabolic rate.

Figure 5.2 shows that any kind of exercise increases the body's energy needs. By monitoring a person running on a treadmill, we can measure the amount of energy the body uses in controlled conditions. Such

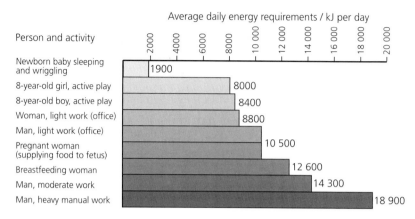

Figure 5.2 Average daily energy requirements of different categories of people undertaking different forms of activity.

measurements help to establish the relationship between energy used and food energy required to fuel our everyday activities. When the energy that the body uses is the same as the intake of food energy, then body weight remains constant.

5.7 Effects of exercise on lung performance

At rest, the lungs have enormous reserves which enable them to meet the greatly increased demands for gaseous exchange during exercise. For example, oxygen consumption of around 500 ml per minute can increase to about 3000 ml per minute in a moderately fit person who is exercising.

A treadmill or stationary bicycle can be used to study the effects of exercise on the volume of air flowing through the lungs (**ventilation**). Figure 5.3 shows that work rate (power) is used as a measure of the level at which a person is exercising. Notice that with increasing work rate, ventilation increases proportionately, but that above a certain work rate it increases more rapidly. At this point oxygen cannot reach the muscles fast enough to supply their needs, in spite of rapid breathing and strenuous pumping of the heart. The muscle cells switch from **aerobic** respiration to **anaerobic** respiration, and the lactic acid produced stimulates increased ventilation.

Exercise also affects other aspects of lung performance. The capacity of the lungs for gaseous exchange improves because of increases in the:

- permeability of lung membranes to the diffusion of gases;
- volume of blood in the capillary blood vessels supplying lung tissue.

These changes occur because exercise distends the blood capillaries. As a result the diffusing capacity of the lungs may increase three-fold.

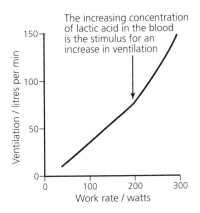

Figure 5.3 The relationship between ventilation and work rate.

Exercise and diabetes

Diabetes is characterised by abnormally high levels of blood sugar due to a reduction in the amount or effectiveness of the hormone **insulin**. Heart disease is common in people with diabetes (**diabetics**) though it is not clear why. Reasons suggested include:

- increased occurrence of hypertension (page 46);
- increased occurrence of obesity (page 42);
- reduced fibrinolysis (page 35);
- increased tendency for platelets to stick together (page 39).

Exercise affects all of these risk factors, as we have seen, by helping reduce weight, beneficially changing blood fat levels and reducing the tendency of the blood to clot. It also helps control blood sugar levels by reducing the body's demand for insulin. Exercise, therefore, has an important part to play in the management of diabetes.

5.8   Effects of exercise on stress

What is stressful to one person is not so to another, and this makes it difficult to define stress. Personality seems to be important – some people are ambitious, competitive and try to cram as much as possible into the time available. They are called **type A** personalities. Their opposites are **type Bs** who are more relaxed and easy going, taking crises calmly in their stride. Research shows that type A people have higher levels of stress hormones like adrenaline in their blood. These hormones raise blood pressure and cholesterol levels which can lead to increased risk of heart disease.

A study of men who worked for the Western Electric Company, USA, showed that type A people also tend to imagine threats from others and feel angry and hostile towards them. Anger is stressful. If we try to accept that our working conditions and the people we work with cannot always be changed and try to divert our stress into other channels, then effective stress management is more likely.

Having a more relaxed attitude to life is one way of managing stress – another is to spend time exercising. People who exercise regularly frequently report a sense of well-being. Vigorous exercise may even produce 'highs'. It seems that exercise stimulates the release of brain chemicals called **endorphins** which have a chemical structure similar to **opium** and **morphine** (page 112). These drugs are addictive, and it is possible that individuals who experience exercise 'highs' are addicted to their own endorphins. Some people who discontinue regular exercise may become irritable, depressed and have disturbed sleep patterns – symptoms similar to those experienced by people withdrawing from addictive drugs.

Exercise, therefore, may reduce stress by altering the secretion of endorphins. However, changes in brain biochemistry are probably not the whole story. For example, not everyone who exercises regularly experiences exercise 'highs', leading some scientists to suggest alternative explanations. For example, exercise 'highs' could be caused by adrenaline or changes in blood gases due to overbreathing when people exert themselves. Whatever the explanation, there seems to be little doubt that exercise contributes to stress control and increases a person's general sense of well-being.

S I X

Food and health

Our diet is the food we eat and drink. It is one of the most important environmental factors affecting health. However, links between diet and health problems are not always clear cut. It is often difficult to pin down *cause and effect*. Rather, different dietary factors are *associated* with particular diseases. For example, a high fat diet is associated with the development of heart disease (chapter 4). However, we are not sure that it *causes* heart disease, even though it seems highly likely that this is the case.

6.1 Basic principles

We need food because the body needs the **nutrients** and energy that food contains. Nutrients are substances necessary for health and growth. Table 6.1 lists the categories of nutrients and their functions in the body. Water is also essential and accounts for about two-thirds of body weight. It is a solvent in which the chemical reactions of metabolism take place and in which substances are transported around the body.

Notice that each category of nutrient performs one or more of three basic functions:

- provides energy – carbohydrates and fats (proteins only when carbohydrates and fats are in short supply);
- serves as components of body structures, and for growth and repair – proteins, minerals and water;
- regulates metabolism – minerals and vitamins.

Gram for gram, the oxidation of protein releases more energy (22.2 kJ per g) than carbohydrate (17.2 kJ per g). Protein is not normally used as an energy source because it is a major component for 'building' the body and for growth and repair. However, when carbohydrates and fats are in short supply, protein is used as an energy source. As a result, muscle wasting may occur.

Table 6.1. Nutrients and their functions in the body

Nutrient	Function
Carbohydrate ⎱ Fat ⎰	Energy stored in carbohydrate and fat molecules is released in the oxidation reactions of cellular respiration. The energy released drives the processes of life.
Protein	Normally, protein is a major source of materials for growth and repair. It is an important component of muscle and all other body tissues.
Minerals	Calcium and phosphorus are major components of bones and teeth. Sodium, potassium and chlorine maintain the osmotic balance of body fluids and are essential for the transmission of nerve impulses. Different minerals regulate metabolism.
Vitamins	Different vitamins regulate metabolism.

The source of nutrients does not affect their role in the body. For example, vitamin C synthesised in the laboratory and taken as a supplement is chemically identical to vitamin C found in oranges. However, the vitamin C supplement does not contain the range of other nutrients found in oranges. These include carbohydrates, B vitamins and different minerals.

Vitamin C regulates different aspects of metabolism by:
- accepting the hydrogen atoms released when amino acids combine to form protein;
- promoting iron absorption in the intestine by converting Fe^{2+}, which is poorly absorbed, to Fe^{3+}, which is readily absorbed;
- acting as an antioxidant, protecting other molecules from types of oxidation reaction that can have harmful consequences.

6.2 Fibre

Fibre is not usually thought of as a nutrient, although it is an important part of our diet. It comes in two forms:
- **Insoluble fibre**, which 'holds' water and swells, but does not dissolve. Seeds and the husks of wheat, rice and other whole grains are important sources of insoluble fibre.

- **Soluble fibre**, which forms a gel-like solution when mixed with water. Fruit pulps, vegetables, oat bran and dried beans are important sources of soluble fibre.

Insoluble fibre adds bulk to food so that the muscles of the intestine can work against it. As a result, food passes through the intestine more quickly. This means that disease-causing substances present in the food and produced by intestinal bacteria do not linger in the intestine.

Soluble fibre slows the absorption of glucose, cholesterol and some minerals through the intestinal wall. High levels of cholesterol are associated with the development of heart disease (chapter 4). With its high content of soluble fibre, oatmeal porridge therefore helps reduce the absorption of cholesterol, perhaps accounting for the increasing popularity of porridge with people who want to lower their blood cholesterol level.

6.3   Towards a healthy diet

We are bombarded with advice on whether or not particular types of food are nutritionally good or bad. 'Experts' tell us that some foods are healthy and others are not. In fact, any food item on its own is 'unhealthy', because no single food contains all of the nutrients in the proportions we need for healthy living. The nutritional value of a particular food depends on the rest of our diet.

A diet that contains nutrients and fibre in the correct amounts and proportions for good health is said to be **balanced** or complete. The idea of four basic **food groups** has been developed to help people choose a balanced diet. Each food group has some nutritional deficiences which are made up by the other three. For example, beef and wholemeal bread lack vitamins A, C and D and are low in calcium. Beef also lacks dietary fibre, which wheat provides. Wheat lacks vitamin B_{12}, which beef provides. Together, beef and wholemeal bread provide more nutrients than either on its own. If fruit and vegetables are added, then vitamins A and C are brought into the diet. Milk and cheese add vitamin D and calcium.

A food that provides appreciable amounts of a range of nutrients but is not energy rich is said to be **nutrient dense**. Fruits, vegetables, bread, cereals, lean meats and milk are examples of nutrient-dense foods. They contribute much more to a balanced diet than so-called **empty-calorie** foods which are energy rich but provide few nutrients (figure 6.1).

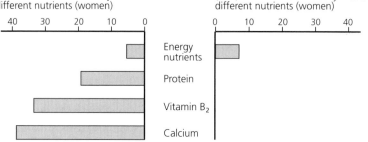

Nutrient-dense food

% contribution of 250 cm³ of skimmed milk to recommended daily intake of different nutrients (women)

Empty-calorie food

% contribution of 250 cm³ of soft drink (cola) to recommended daily intake of different nutrients (women)

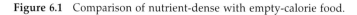

Figure 6.1 Comparison of nutrient-dense with empty-calorie food.

6.4 Diet during pregnancy

During pregnancy, a woman's nutritional needs change. Extra nutrients are needed for the developing fetus and placenta. Blood volume increases, the lining of the uterus thickens and the breasts enlarge. Extra fat is laid down, mostly on the hips and thighs. Different components of the weight gained during pregnancy are shown in table 6.2.

The total extra energy needs of a pregnant woman amount to around 0.8 MJ per day more than the 9 MJ per day recommended for the typical non-pregnant woman. Increases in the efficiency of insulin-controlled glucose metabolism and nutrient absorption meet the extra demand, so

Table 6.2. Typical weight gain during pregnancy

Component	Mass/kg
Fetus	3.6
Uterus	0.9
Placenta	0.7
Maternal blood	2.0
Amniotic fluid	0.9
Breast tissue	0.4
Fat tissue	3.9
Tissue fluid	1.1
Total weight gain	13.5

for most nutrients the small additional amounts needed are covered adequately by the woman's normal diet – there is no need for her to eat more. However, for a few nutrients, intake during pregnancy is more critical.

Folate

Folate (folic acid) is a vitamin which activates enzymes that control DNA replication and protein synthesis. It is therefore particularly important for growth. Low folate intake during pregnancy may cause abnormal growth of the fetus. In particular, folate deficiency is associated with developmental abnormalities of the spinal cord such as **spina bifida** (failure of the neural tube to close). Foods rich in folate include liver, kidney, wholegrain cereals and dark green vegetables. Such food items are often not a regular part of the pregnant woman's diet, which is why supplements of around 0.4 mg of folate a day are recommended during pregnancy.

Calcium

Calcium uptake by the fetus is especially high during the last three months of pregnancy when its bones are mineralising. The calcium normally comes from the mother's diet, though if dietary sources are low, calcium is drawn from the mother's bones, especially the long bones of the arms and legs. This ensures that the fetus obtains as much calcium as it needs, even if the mother's diet contains little of it. Supplementation therefore aims to benefit the mother rather than protect the fetus, and recommended intake of calcium during pregnancy is 1200 mg a day. Increasing the intake of milk and cheese is the easiest way of obtaining the extra calcium needed (0.5 litres of milk and 60 g of Cheddar cheese each supply about 600 mg of calcium).

Iron

Iron deficiency is common in pregnant women. During pregnancy, a woman's iron requirements are raised due to increases in haemoglobin synthesis and storage of iron by the fetus. Foods rich in iron include meat (especially liver), whole grains and prunes, but even if her diet regularly includes these items, it can be difficult for a pregnant woman to obtain enough iron from food alone.

Pregnant women who develop iron deficiency may deliver infants that are small and at risk from developing iron deficiency in their first year. Many doctors, therefore, recommend iron supplementation at around 30 mg a day. However, iron supplements can cause constipation, and excessive amounts of iron (more than 100 mg a day) decrease zinc absorption and may cause zinc deficiency.

Zinc

Zinc is an important component of enzymes that control DNA and protein synthesis. Normal growth, therefore, depends on an adequate supply of zinc, and zinc deficiency is associated with the delivery of small infants that may have growth abnormalities. The recommended intake of zinc during pregnancy is 15 mg a day, and studies show that many pregnant women fail to meet the recommended level in their diet. Zinc supplementation does not seem to help, so the intake of foods rich in zinc is encouraged. Oysters are very rich in zinc, though this source is perhaps not so appealing as others which include red meats, beans, peas, whole grains and milk – all of which are also good sources of other nutrients. Limiting iron supplements to 30 mg a day also helps to reduce the threat of zinc deficiency (see above).

The nausea and vomiting that many pregnant women experience is called **morning sickness** (although it can occur at any time of the day). The symptoms are related to hormonal changes, especially during the first three months of pregnancy. Daily doses of 5–10 mg of vitamin B_6 relieve the condition in some, but not all, cases.

6.5 Infant feeding

Newborn infants depend on others to feed them, and for their first few months are fed only one food – milk. The nutritional quality of the milk is therefore critical. The nutrient composition of milks from different species varies because the young of each species have particular nutritional needs that depend on their rate of growth, metabolism and ability to digest different substances. Human infants, for example, grow slowly and are born with an immature digestive system. Human milk contains more carbohydrate and less vitamins than, for example, cow's milk.

The breast milk a mother produces during the first few days after giving birth is called **colostrum**. It contains more protein, minerals and antibodies than the milk produced later. The antibodies help protect the infant from infections and allergies as it adjusts from the germ-free environment of the womb to the world outside. The milk produced later is called **mature** milk. It consists of:

- **foremilk**, which collects in the milk ducts connecting the milk-producing cells of the breast to the nipple;
- **hindmilk**, which is produced and stored in the milk-producing cells.

Foremilk contains more carbohydrate and protein than hindmilk. The infant receives foremilk when feeding begins; hindmilk becomes available only when it is ejected from the nipple through the action of the hormone **oxytocin** on the milk-producing cells. This is known as the **let-down reflex**. Hindmilk contains much more fat than foremilk and helps satisfy the infant's hunger. Failure of the let-down reflex (see box) is a major reason why some mothers are not able to breastfeed properly. The infant is hungry much of the time and growth and development may suffer.

> The **let-down reflex** releases hindmilk. The infant's sucking on the nipple stimulates neural pathways from the brain to the **pituitary gland**. Oxytocin is released from the pituitary into the mother's blood and circulates to the breast where it causes the milk-producing cells to contract and release their contents.

Although breast milk is ideal for infant feeding, 'formula' milks used for bottle-feeding are close to human breast milk in composition. Most formula milks are based on modified cow's milk (table 6.3).

 Breast milk is sweeter than formula milk, although infants appear to like the taste of both. What a mother eats affects the composition of breast milk (see below) and therefore its taste. How such early experiences of taste influence our food preferences later in life is not clear, though some scientists claim that they can affect our choice of diet and therefore our health during adulthood. It seems that healthy eating may begin at birth!

Table 6.3. Comparison of human breast milk, cow's milk and commercial formula milk

Nutrient	Human milk	Cow's milk	Formula milk (diluted)
Carbohydrate/g	7.4	5.0	7.2
Fat/g	4.2	3.7	3.6
Protein/g	1.1	3.5	1.5
Calcium/mg	35.0	120.0	49.0
Phosphorus/mg	15.0	95.0	30.0
Iron/mg	0.075	0.05	0.9
Vitamin C/mg	3.8	1.5	6.9
Vitamin D/mg	0.8	0.15	1.1

Nutrient values are per 100 cm^3.

Diet and breastfeeding

Breast milk production depends on how often the infant feeds and how much he or she takes at each feed. About 850 cm^3 of milk is a good daily average. To meet this demand, a breastfeeding woman needs an extra 25% energy intake each day.

Fat stored during pregnancy meets some of the energy needs during breastfeeding, and increased food intake accounts for the rest (breastfeeding women are normally more hungry than usual and therefore eat more). Extra nutrients are also needed, most of which come with the extra energy intake, providing the diet is varied and taken from each of the four basic food groups. However, calcium, folate, iron and vitamin D may be in short supply. A daily litre of milk can provide the extra calcium; iron supplement helps replace the stores of iron lost during pregnancy (page 61); and vitamin D supplement is recommended for those mothers who are exposed to little sunshine and who are vegetarian.

Because the milk-producing cells in the breast use raw materials from the mother's blood, what a mother eats affects the composition of her milk. Although the amounts of carbohydrate, protein and fat in breast milk vary little in response to the mother's diet, the vitamin content and the amounts of several minerals do. For example, beri beri (thiamin deficiency) and pernicious anaemia (vitamin B$_{12}$ deficiency) may occur in infants of mothers deficient in these vitamins; infants that do not receive enough zinc and iodine grow and develop slowly. Mothers should aim for a varied and balanced diet as the best way of achieving good nutrition during breastfeeding, rather than relying on vitamin and mineral supplements.

Substances other than nutrients can enter breast milk. For example, a breastfeeding infant receives a small dose of caffeine when his or her mother drinks a cup of coffee. Alcohol also passes into the breast milk if the mother drinks beer, wine or spirits. Neither caffeine nor alcohol pose a threat to the infant, providing the mother moderates her intake. However, tremors develop in infants exposed to too much caffeine (if the mother drinks 10 or more cups per day), and development of the brain and nervous system is retarded in cases of excess alcohol (if the mother drinks 6 or more units per day).

Almost any drug in the mother's blood will enter the breast milk. For most drugs the infant receives less than 1% of the mother's dose without ill effect. Some drugs, however, are concentrated in the milk and should not be taken by a breastfeeding woman. Certain poisons may also be transferred via breast milk. For example, environmental pollutants such as PCBs (waste products of various industrial processes) and the insecticides DDT and chlordane are fat soluble. If ingested in food they may be stored in a woman's fat tissues. Later on, when the fat stores are used in milk production, the pollutants pass into her milk. Infants exposed to these substances may develop rashes and problems with the nervous system and digestion.

6.6 Diet for children

Children are not miniature adults and their diet should match their needs for energy and nutrients, which are different from those of adults. Such needs are greatest in very young children because they are growing rapidly and have a high basal metabolic rate (page 53). For example, weight for weight a 4-month-old infant needs to take in three times more energy than a 30-year-old adult. This means that assuming the infant takes in nearly 17% of his or her body weight in milk each day, an adult weighing 70 kg and also taking in 17% of his or her body weight in milk would need to drink 16 litres of it a day!

Growth occurs whenever cells in the body increase in number or in size. Each tissue and organ has its own **critical period** for growth. For example, the critical period for the brain is during fetal development and the first year after birth; for muscle tissue, bone and fat tissue the critical periods are during infancy and adolescence. An adequate supply of nutrients needed for growth during the critical periods helps avoid setbacks in development.

Developmental progress is most easily followed by measuring height and weight regularly through childhood and adolescence. Figure 6.2 summarises average yearly growth in height and weight for girls and boys together with the changes in their average energy and nutrient requirements.

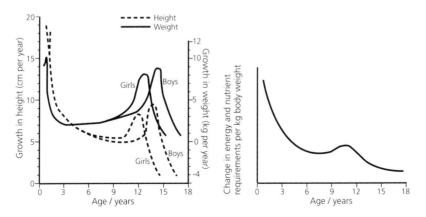

Figure 6.2 Changes in height, weight, and energy and nutrient requirements during childhood and adolescence.

Current UK dietary advice recommends that breast/bottle-feeding should continue for the first six months of life. Soft, solid food may be added to the diet of milk between the ages of four and six months. Infant rice cereal fortified with iron is usually the first item to be introduced, then strained vegetables and fruits. In the weeks that follow, the infant can start on other single-ingredient foods, one at a time half-weekly. The interval between the introduction of each new food gives time for the recognition of symptoms should an allergic response or intolerance to a particular food develop. Infants can move on to cut-up and mashed adult foods after the age of 12 months or earlier.

Breast milk, formula milks and commercially prepared infant food are nutritionally complete. Most infants, therefore, do not need vitamin or mineral supplements. However, vitamin D supplement is recommended for infants that spend little time in the sunshine or whose diet is vitamin D deficient. Also, in areas where drinking water is not fluoridated, fluoride tablets or drops are an insurance against the development of dental caries.

Food allergy occurs when a food substance acts as antigens, stimulating the body to develop an immune response (chapter 2). The abnormally high blood levels of the antibodies produced against the antigenic food substance help to identify it. Wheat, gluten, egg white protein and cow's milk protein are common food antigens (hence infant cereals are based on rice rather than wheat). Symptoms of food allergy include diarrhoea, rashes, a runny nose (**rhinitis**) and irritated eyes.

Food intolerance, on the other hand, does not involve the immune system. Food substances affecting digestive processes are often the cause. For example, **lactose intolerance** occurs in people that lack the enzyme **lactase** which digests the sugar. Bacteria in the intestine feed on the undigested lactose, excreting fatty acids and gases which produce symptoms such as diarrhoea and stomach cramps. Milk contains lactose, though lactase-deficient people may be able to tolerate cheese, yoghurt and other milk products because processing partly breaks down the lactose.

Eating patterns through childhood are largely controlled by the home environment. Between the ages of one and four years the growth rate slows and children of these ages may be less enthusiastic about food than during their first year. Also, food likes and dislikes develop depending on how and what foods are offered. Anxious parents may try to coax children to eat more and try out a more varied diet. However, providing a child's diet consists of different items chosen from each of the four basic food groups in sufficient quantities, and he or she is growing normally and remains healthy, then there is little cause for concern.

Eating patterns often change dramatically during adolescence. Busy with school and friends and establishing their individual identity, teenagers may not eat regular meals. Increased appetites, especially during growth 'spurts', may be satisfied by 'snacking' through the day. Although many of the foods may be nutritionally poor, the sheer volume eaten helps most adolescents meet their energy and nutrient needs.

Diet during childhood and adolescence affects present and future health. Insufficient intake of energy nutrients, protein, iron or zinc slows growth and results in underweight individuals vulnerable to infectious diseases. Excess energy intake produces overweight individuals, especially when levels of physical activity are low.

The types of food selected from the food groups is important. Wholegrain bread and cereals should be included, and boiled, baked and steamed foods should be eaten more often than fried foods. For example, hamburgers, chips and other fast foods are often high in fat. Also, the bun around the hamburger may be low in fibre. Although many fast foods fit into the basic food groups, a fast-food diet is likely to be unbalanced (page 59) – high in fat, low in fibre and deficient in minerals and vitamins (especially calcium and vitamins A and C). Sufficient calcium for bone formation is particularly important. During growth 'spurts' as much as 10 g of calcium per year accumulates in the skeleton. A poor diet may also lead to iron deficiency in adolescent girls who are menstruating. Girls who diet because they are unhappy with their 'image' may also be deficient in iron and other nutrients. In some cases, dieting leads to **anorexia nervosa**, whose treatment usually requires the skills of a psychotherapist and dietitian.

Around 85% of adolescents suffer at some time from **acne**. Pimples form when bacteria enter through the skin and cause local infection underneath. Because acne develops beneath the skin, the pimples cannot be washed away or prevented easily by good hygiene. Creams containing antibiotics, benzoyl peroxide and, in severe cases, vitamin A-like drugs are effective treatments but may produce side effects such as itchiness, headaches and raised cholesterol levels. Little evidence supports the popular belief that acne is aggravated by eating sweets, fatty foods and other 'unhealthy' food items.

6.7 Diet for adults

Because the effects of nutrition on health develop over the long-term, diet-related diseases tend to emerge in older adults. Other factors such as smoking, life-style and biological ageing also combine to affect the rate of appearance of disease. Reduced physical activity, muscle mass and metabolic rate result in decreased energy needs, but requirements for protein, calcium and vitamins A and D may increase. During adulthood, therefore, the focus should shift from diets that promote growth to ones that maintain health.

The adult diet should contain a wide variety of foods from the basic food groups. Unsaturates should be the primary source of fat, cholesterol intake should be less than 300 mg per day, sodium intake may need to be reduced and high fibre foods should be eaten in preference to highly refined alternatives. Recommended amounts (expressed as percentages) for different energy sources are shown in table 6.4. British and American recommendations for the adult diet are the same, despite being prepared by different committees and taking into account a wide variety of views on diet. They are summarised in table 6.5. More regular exercise is an important addition to this programme.

Elderly people should continue to follow the dietary recommendation for younger adults. In addition:

- small daily doses of vitamin D (5–10 mg a day) are recommended for the housebound and those who spend most of their time indoors;
- women should maintain a good daily intake of calcium from low-fat milk, cheese and other milk products. This may help reduce the risk of calcium loss from bones (osteoporosis) – page 18 ;
- regular portions of fatty fish or small doses of fish oil may reduce the risk of thrombosis (page 39).

Many elderly people have altered their diets to take account of nutritional advice – it is never too late to make changes for the better.

Table 6.4. Recommended contribution of energy nutrients to adult diet

Energy nutrient	% Total energy
Carbohydrate	55
Fat	30
Protein	15

Table 6.5. Average British and American recommendations for the adult diet

Eat less	Eat more
Alcohol	Wholegrain cereals
Sugar	Vegetables
Fat	Fruit
Salt	

6.8 Malnutrition

Malnutrition literally means 'poor nutrition'. When there is not enough food, children do not grow at the normal rate, and children and adults lose weight. Worldwide, being underweight is one of the major risks to health. People of developing countries who live in slums and shanty towns are especially at risk. Food at affordable prices and clean drinking water are often in short supply.

Pregnant women, breastfeeding women and growing children have a greater need for food than other people. Children, in particular, need energy for growth and good health. Energy-starved children fail to grow at the normal rate and are more vulnerable to infectious diseases such as measles, tuberculosis and chicken-pox. Deficiency diseases, especially of vitamin A, protein and the minerals zinc and iron, are more likely to develop. Energy shortage also makes children look emaciated ('skin and bones') – a condition called **marasmus**. By contrast, figure 6.3 shows that

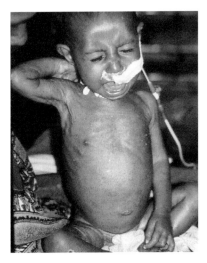

Figure 6.3 The appearance of a child suffering from kwashiorkor.

children who are short of protein may look normal or even fat. Their appearance is due to the accumulation of water – a condition called **kwashiorkor**. In most cases the cure for underweight children and adults is *more* food. This solution to the problem, however, is not easily achieved. Although many countries produce food surpluses, food availability can be erratic.

Poor farming methods coupled with environmental damage can lead to mass starvation. For example, in the Sahel region of West Africa an age-old system of farming developed which was in tune with the environment. Farmers grew sorghum and millet in the wetter south, while nomadic herdsmen in the drier north moved with their cattle from pasture to pasture so as not to overburden the area's ecology – made fragile through low rainfall. In the 1950s and 60s, more and more land was used to grow peanuts for export to earn foreign exchange. During the dry season, the herdsmen were deprived of grazing land for their cattle and the farmers had no natural manure to fertilise their crops. Although artificial fertiliser was available, it was too expensive for the farmers to use.

Increasing debt and declining soil fertility was coupled, in 1969, with a drop in world prices for peanuts. Farmers tried to maintain their living standards by growing more peanuts further north toward the semi-desert used by the nomadic herdsmen. When the rains failed, crops died and disaster struck. More than 100 000 people died in the famine that followed.

Starvation results from lack of food and causes loss of body fat and muscle tissue. A decrease in the heart rate of up to 30% can result in people who are suffering from starvation feeling cold, even in warm conditions. There are also psychological effects – poor concentration, irritability, disturbed sleep and preoccupation with food are some of the experiences of people deprived of food long term.

In developed countries, some people are underweight through slimming but relatively few because of malnutrition. Excess food is the much more common form of malnutrition. If a person eats more than is necessary for his or her energy needs, the excess is turned into fat which is stored in fat cells under the skin, and he or she puts on weight.

The health implications of being overweight include an increased risk of heart disease, stroke, arthritis and diabetes. Treatment aims to reduce the intake of food energy *gradually*. 'Crash' diets almost never work, the initial weight loss being mostly water. Few people are able to stick to a diet that demands major upheavals in their eating habits, and the weight soon goes back on. A diet consisting of a variety of nutrient-dense (page 59) foods chosen from the four basic food groups and eaten regularly in modest amounts slowly brings about weight reduction and also helps maintain it. Increased exercise helps as well. The aim is to alter a person's exercise and eating habits gradually. It is much easier to adjust to modest changes such as eating smaller amounts of food and using stairs instead of lifts than to make sudden, drastic changes.

Oral rehydration therapy

Victims of diarrhoea lose water because food and water are not absorbed through the gut wall. Giving patients a solution of table salt and sugar saves thousands of lives daily worldwide. Figure 6.4 shows how the treatment works. Membrane-bound protein carrier molecules in the cells lining the gut accept sodium and glucose simultaneously. The carrier molecules transfer the sodium into the gut cells. Another membrane-bound protein molecule then pumps out the sodium into the extracellular fluid surrounding the gut cells. The high levels of extracellular sodium draw water from the gut by osmosis. Treatment of patients with glucose/sodium chloride powder in solution improves the body's water retention by up to 25 times. Children close to death through the dehydration caused by diarrhoea can recover within a few hours of treatment.

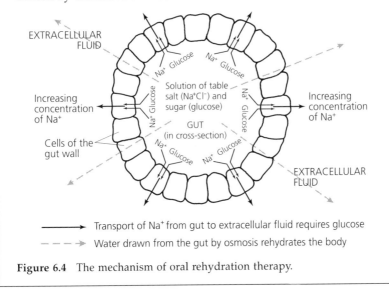

Figure 6.4 The mechanism of oral rehydration therapy.

SEVEN

Diseases of the gaseous exchange system

A sneeze produces a jet of moisture droplets from the nose and mouth. Microorganisms infecting the mucous membranes lining the nose and rest of the **upper respiratory tract** (pharynx, larynx, trachea and bronchi) are carried in the droplets to other people nearby. This is how diseases like **colds** and **influenza (flu)** pass from person to person, especially in crowded places like schools and hospitals.

Figure 7.1 shows the virus that causes flu. The projections from the surface of the virus are proteins which bind the virus to the cells of the mucous membrane and help the virus to penetrate it. The infected cells are destroyed, and within 48 hours the symptoms of flu develop. Muscles ache and overproduction of mucus causes a runny nose, sneezing and coughing. A sore throat and fever develop, and the patient feels generally unwell. The symptoms are caused by the virus stimulating production of **interferon** by the virus-infected cells. Interferon is a protein which helps healthy cells break down viruses and prevent them from multiplying.

Symptoms of flu usually subside within 2–7 days unless the infection spreads to the lungs. Then viral **pneumonia** may set in making the patient seriously ill. The lungs fill with liquid, and bacteria may set up other infections.

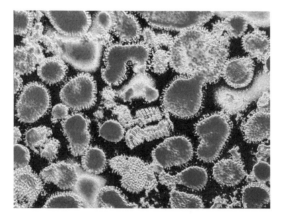

Figure 7.1 Electronmicrograph of flu viruses.

Pneumonia is also caused by a particular type of bacterium. The patient becomes breathless because the liquid which accumulates in the lungs reduces the surface area of the alveoli available for the absorption of oxygen. Bacteria can also infect the **pleural membranes** which line the ribcage and cover the surfaces of the lungs. The infection, called **pleurisy**, roughens the membranes causing pain when they rub together during breathing.

The surface proteins of the flu virus are antigens against which an infected person produces antibodies (page 24). However, people may catch flu more than once during their lifetime. Frequent viral mutations are the problem as these can result in changes in antigen shape. Minor changes are called **antigenic drifts**. They produce new *strains* of virus which are probably responsible for the frequent occurrence of flu epidemics. Major changes are called **antigenic shifts** and result in new *types* of virus. They are less frequent than antigenic drifts and seem to be linked to the 10–20-year cycle of worldwide pandemics. The occurrence of antigenic drift and antigenic shift means that antibodies produced against a particular type of flu virus do not protect the person from a new infection. It also means that producing an effective vaccine is difficult.

The World Health Organisation monitors the antigenic changes in flu viruses and recommends the strains of virus which should be included in vaccines. Protective immunisation is usually given to young children, the elderly and other people who are particularly at risk from flu. Protection from a particular strain of flu virus is effective providing the vaccine for the strain is given each year and that its antigens do not change. When antigenic changes occur, the vaccine is redeveloped quickly to keep pace.

Other respiratory infections are classified according to the region of the upper respiratory tract affected:

- infection of the throat (pharynx) is called **pharyngitis**;
- infection of the voicebox (larynx) is called **laryngitis**;
- infection of the windpipe (trachea) is called **tracheitis**;
- infection of the bronchi and bronchioles is called **bronchitis**.

Treating patients suffering from viral infections amounts to little more than bed rest and good care. Very few drugs are effective against viral diseases, including flu, although **amantidine** is available for patients who are at risk of serious illness. This drug seems to prevent the flu virus from reproducing in the cells of the mucous membrane. A person who is ill with flu is susceptible to attack by bacteria. Infections caused by bacteria are treated with antibiotics (page 138).

Other diseases, like **lung cancer** and **asthma** are not caused by bacteria and viruses. Lung cancer is caused by a number of factors but most commonly by smoking cigarettes (pages 74 and 127). Asthma, in which the victim finds it difficult to breathe, is often caused by allergies. The occurrence of lung cancer and asthma can be linked to air quality.

7.1 Smoking and lung cancer: making the link

The ways in which substances in tobacco smoke affect health are discussed in chapters 4 and 11. Here we are concerned with data that link smoking with lung cancer.

Figure 7.2 shows the sort of evidence which alerted scientists to a possible correlation between smoking cigarettes and lung cancer. Deaths from the disease increased sharply from the early 1900s when deaths from other forms of lung disease (in this case pulmonary tuberculosis, page 4) were falling. At the time the habit of smoking cigarettes was newly established and widespread. Although it was difficult to prove the link irrefutably, many doctors who saw the evidence understood its significance. Many of them gave up smoking cigarettes with the result that the occurrence of lung cancer among doctors went down compared with the population as a whole. Other studies established clearly the relationship between the risk of dying from lung cancer and the number of cigarettes smoked – the more cigarettes smoked, the greater the risk (figure 7.3).

Cigarette smoking is also the cause of another disease called **emphysema** (figure 7.4). The substances in tobacco smoke stimulate cells (called **mast cells**) in the lungs to produce proteolytic (protein-digesting) enzymes. These enzymes break down the walls of the alveoli creating enlarged chambers. The surface area of the lungs available for the absorption of oxygen is therefore decreased. Oxygenation of the blood is reduced with the result that even a small increase in physical effort makes the victim of emphysema breathless and exhausted.

Illnesses caused by cigarette smoking represent a major challenge for preventative medicine, and the campaign against smoking has been fought hard. Cigarette sales have fluctuated, but the overall trend is downward. Evidence suggests that non-smokers also suffer increased risks of ill health when they breathe in smoke from other people's cigarettes – so-called **passive smoking,** and this has lent support to the assertion that people have the right to a smoke-free environment. Smoking is now banned in many public places. Between 1972 and 1984 cigarette smoking in Britain dropped by almost a third. Today, there are twice as many non-smokers as smokers.

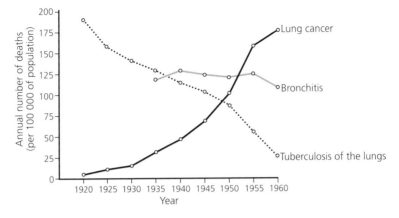

Figure 7.2 Deaths from lung disease in England and Wales, 1920–60.

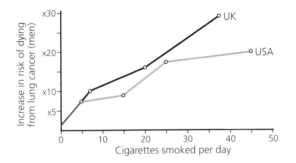

Figure 7.3 The relationship between the risk of dying from lung cancer and the number of cigarettes smoked daily (men).

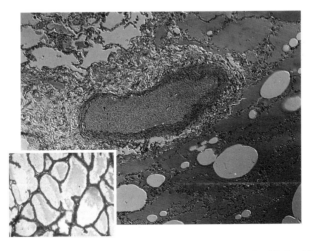

Figure 7.4 Alveoli destroyed by emphysema, compared with healthy lung tissue (*inset*).

7.2 Asthma

In Britain, respiratory diseases account for around 33 million lost working days each year, representing about 9% of all days lost through illness. Of these lost days, about 6 million are attributable to asthma.

What is asthma?

Asthma is a common condition characterised by obstruction to the flow of air through the airways of the upper respiratory tract. Attacks of wheezing, difficulty with breathing and a feeling of tightness in the chest are symptoms often experienced by people suffering from asthma. In mild cases of asthma, symptoms only appear from time to time, but in more severe cases airflow never completely returns to normal between attacks. Obstruction to the flow of air is due to narrowing of the airways resulting from inflammation. In severe cases, plugs of mucus may block the airways, obstructing airflow further.

Diagnosing asthma

A doctor confronted by a person complaining of the symptoms listed above should at least suspect that the person is asthmatic. Showing that airflow is obstructed confirms the diagnosis. The data for diagnosis is obtained using a **spirometer**.

A patient linked up to the equipment breathes out (exhales) as hard as possible after breathing in (inhaling) as completely as he or she can. The volume of air exhaled in the first second is called the **peak volume**

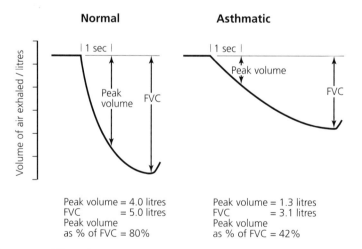

Figure 7.5 Effect of asthma on peak volume as a percentage of forced vital capacity (FVC).

and the total volume exhaled is the **forced vital capacity (FVC)**. Normally, peak volume is about 80% of FVC. However, figure 7.5 shows that the percentage is much lower in asthmatics. Vigorous exercise highlights this effect, helping diagnosis. If peak flow and FVC immediately following 10 minutes of running are more than 15% below the values recorded before exercise began, this strongly suggests that the person undertaking the test is asthmatic.

Causes of asthma

Around 10% of children aged 5 to 12 years suffer from asthma – young boys more so than young girls. Some children improve during the teenage years and grow out of the problem by the time they are in their early twenties. However, different studies indicate that there is a slow increase in the prevalence of the disease in most countries.

In some families there is evidence of a genetic link for asthma which can be traced through previous generations. However, different factors in the environment seem to be the main triggers of asthma attacks (table 7.1). It seems that the immune system of vulnerable individuals responding to different environmental antigens (figure 2.5) causes the inflammation of the airways observed in asthma patients.

Table 7.1.   Environmental triggers of asthma

Environmental factor	Effect
Exercise	Narrows airways and can be used as a diagnostic test for asthma. Swimming in an indoor heated pool is least likely to cause an attack; running in cold, dry air is more likely to provoke an asthmatic response.
House dust mites	A source of antigens (page 22) which can cause inflammation of the airways. Mites are widely distributed in bedding, soft furnishing, carpets and soft toys.
Pollen and spores	A source of antigens causing seasonal asthma when the pollen count is high. Attacks are usually associated with grass pollens, which are most common in June and July. Mould spores are widespread in July and August.
Pets	Antigens which trigger asthma are present in cats' fur, saliva and urine. *cont.*

Table 7.1. *continued*

Environmental factor	Effect
Occupation	Jobs which expose people to certain substances can trigger asthma attacks in vulnerable individuals. 'Problem' substances include hair sprays, wood dust, coffee beans and various drugs.
Food	Various foods may cause non-asthma allergic responses in some people. However some foodstuffs, especially milk, eggs, nuts and wheat, may cause asthma attacks in vulnerable individuals.
Drugs	Beta blockers (page 48) and aspirin are those that are mostly responsible for cases of drug-induced asthma.
Pollution	Poor air quality (high levels of ozone, sulphur dioxide, oxides of nitrogen and dust particles) provokes narrowing of the airways and may trigger asthma attacks.

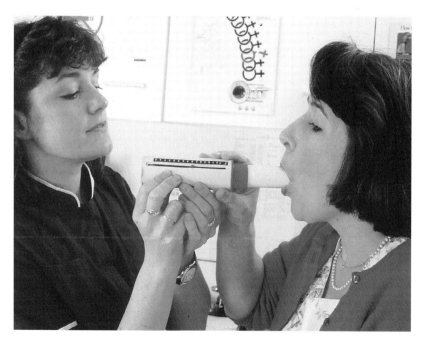

Figure 7.6 Using a peak flow meter.

Treating asthma

The speed of onset of asthma attacks varies. Symptoms may appear within a few minutes without warning or develop slowly over days or weeks. Testing peak flow at home using a **peak flow meter** (figure 7.6) helps to monitor the situation. The most common symptoms are breathlessness and increasing difficulty with inhalation. Mild attacks are controlled with **bronchodilators** – drugs that dilate (widen) the airways.

ß-adrenergic agonists (page 112) are the best and safest bronchodilators. Examples are salbutamol and terbutaline. The drugs are fast acting and when, for example, taken by asthmatic children 15–20 minutes before exercise help prevent wheezing. Salmeterol is another example of a bronchodilator. Its effects last longer than other agonists and the drug is particularly suitable for preventing night-time symptoms of asthma which may develop while a child is asleep. Bronchodilators are best inhaled. Different inhalation devices help the patient to breathe in the drug as an aerosol or powder.

A severe attack of asthma is a frightening experience for both children and adults. Reassuring the patient is an important part of coping with the situation. Immediate improvement following treatment with bronchodilators does not always mean that severe symptoms will not return. Continued observation is important, and if the patient does not improve then medical help should be sought immediately.

E I G H T

Kidney failure

A decline in the function of the kidneys is a warning that something is wrong. Fall in urine output, increasingly acidic urine and retention of potassium ions (K^+) in the urine are symptoms which alert the doctor to the possibility of developing kidney failure. Warning signs include:

- impaired concentration, drowsiness and convulsions;
- heart failure;
- nausea and vomiting;
- swollen feet.

A doctor's first task is to distinguish between **acute kidney failure** and **chronic kidney failure**. The symptoms of acute disease are abrupt, short term and, once diagnosed, may be reversible. The symptoms of chronic disease are long term, often irreversible and may require more drastic treatment. In both cases some of the symptoms are the same, making assessment of the condition difficult. However, precise diagnosis is important so that the correct treatment of the patient can begin.

8.1 Acute kidney failure

The causes of acute renal failure fall into three broad categories:

- the blood supply to the kidneys can decrease because of heavy bleeding, infection or loss of fluids as a result of burns or severe diarrhoea;
- thrombosis (page 39), bacterial infection or various drugs can cause structural changes in the nephrons and accumulation of fluid in the kidneys;
- blockage of the collecting ducts or obstruction of the ureter or urethra can be a result of cancer, 'stones' (ureter only) or swelling of the prostate gland (urethra only).

General procedures aim to keep the patient alive while the cause of the acute failure is assessed so that the appropriate treatment can begin. Some of the treatments used to deal with the different causes of acute kidney failure include:

- Improvement of the blood supply to the kidneys by drugs which reverse restriction of the renal vessels. The treatment helps prevent damage to the kidneys and the onset of structural changes in the nephrons. Restricting the intake of sodium (Na^+) and potassium (K^+) helps maintain the ionic composition of the blood at safe levels.

- The use of antibiotic drugs (page 15) to treat bacterial infections which may result because of the reduced efficiency of the immune system (chapter 2). However, because the patient's condition means that excretion of different substances (including drugs) is less than normal, drug dosage has to be kept at a level which avoids possible problems with toxicity.

- The use of ultrasound scanning (page 90) and **computer-assisted tomography** to help visualise blockage of the ureter and urethra. Removal of the obstruction rapidly improves diuresis (urine production) and the prospects of curing the patient.

The different treatments may bring about a rapid increase in diuresis. After this, kidney function gradually improves over a period of months, but rarely returns to normal except in younger patients. Deaths from acute kidney failure are high (around 50% of cases), many of them due to the patient's increased vulnerability to infections.

8.2 Chronic kidney failure

Chronic glomerulonephritis is a common cause of chronic kidney failure. The membranes of the glomerulus begin to leak protein into the urine, whereas normally protein molecules are too large to pass from the blood in the glomerulus to the Bowman's capsule. Because of the loss of protein, the osmotic pressure of the blood falls. The fluid that bathes cells, which normally would pass back into the capillary blood vessels, instead accumulates in the tissues (**oedema**), and 'puffiness' develops – swollen feet is one of the warning signs of chronic kidney failure. The accumulation of tissue fluid is symptomatic and helps a doctor to distinguish between the chronic and acute kidney condition.

Unfortunately, chronic kidney failure is generally incurable. To begin with, mineral supplements (to replace lost sodium and prevent loss of calcium from bones), and strict control of protein and fluid intake aim to delay the progressive deterioration of kidney function. However, all of the glomeruli are eventually affected. When all else fails, more aggressive measures are called for.

Dialysis

A patient with chronic kidney failure may be attached to a kidney machine which removes waste substances from the blood – a process called **haemodialysis**. Figure 8.1 shows how a kidney machine works. Blood is drawn from one of the patient's main veins and passed through the machine. The thin, selectively permeable membrane separates small diffusible molecules (wastes) from large non-diffusible ones (blood proteins) whilst maintaining the correct pH and balance of fluid and ions in the blood.

Most patients require dialysis two or three times a week for 4–8 hours at a time. The majority of patients in the UK are treated at home. After two years, patient survival is around 88%, and eight years later approximately 50% of patients are still alive. Death is usually due to infection or disease of the heart or blood vessels.

Transplantation

A kidney transplant offers the patient freedom from the weekly routine of linking up to a kidney machine. However, the supply of suitable donor kidneys limits the number of transplant operations. Rejection of transplants between unrelated individuals is the major threat, and matching donor with recipient as nearly as possible is crucial to successful treatment. Assessment of the ABO (blood group) antigens (page 32) and human

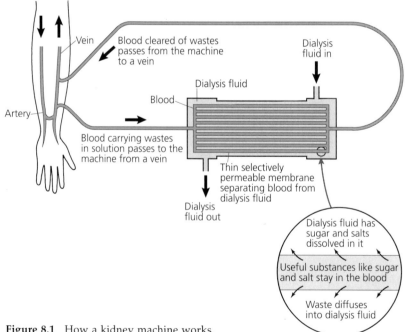

Figure 8.1 How a kidney machine works.

lymphocyte antigens (HLA) (pages 29 and 126) is routine. The antigens coded for by the HLA–A and HLA–B genes produce the strongest rejection reactions. Compatibility between donor and recipient is assessed by the identical match of ABO antigens and HLA–A/HLA–B.

The majority of donor kidneys come from people who have just died. However, it is possible to live a healthy life with only one kidney and the donor may be someone living who wants to help the patient. Live donors are often close relatives of the patient. Their body tissues are more nearly compatible, reducing the chances of rejection by the recipient.

Following transplant surgery, the patient is given immuno-suppressive drugs (page 29) to prevent rejection of the transplanted kidney. The antifungal agent cyclosporine (page 29) has improved the prospects of transplant patients dramatically. The cost of maintaining a transplant patient after the operation is much less than maintaining a patient on dialysis. However, rejection remains a long-term problem. Acute (sudden) rejection usually means the kidney must be removed quickly, and re-implantation with a fresh kidney is an option. If rejection is less sudden, then the patient becomes increasingly unwell. Treatment with drugs may slow (even halt) the process, but the possibility of eventual failure is high.

Fertility and contraception

The **fertility rate** gives the average number of children a woman has throughout her childbearing life. Estimates of the number of births and size of families are an essential part of population projections by which governments plan future economic and social policies. Table 9.1 compares the fertility rates for different European countries.

For each country, notice the fall from 1970 to 1992 in the number of children born per woman and the fall in the birth rate among teenage mothers (although remaining high in the UK). Also notice that, on the whole, fertility rates decline as women get older.

The decline in fertility rates since 1970 is due to a number of factors. On average more women now delay starting their families, and when they do start, they tend to have fewer children. Also, more women are choosing not to have children at all.

Table 9.1. Fertility rates for selected European countries

| | Births per 1000 women | | | | Total fertility rate | |
| | 1970 Age/years | | 1992 Age/years | | | |
Country	15–19	40–44	15–19	40–44	1970	1992
UK	49.1	9.2	31.8	5.5	2.4	1.8
France	26.7	13.6	8.6	7.6	2.5	1.7
Netherlands	17.0	16.8	5.5	5.7	2.6	1.6
Germany	37.4	9.7	13.4	4.5	2.0	1.3
Italy	20.9	19.5	6.1	6.3	2.4	1.3

Source: Office of Population Censuses and Surveys.

9.1 Effects of pregnancy on maternal physiology

The human female usually produces one mature egg each month from the onset of **puberty** (age 11–14 years) to the beginning of the **menopause** (age about 45 years). This monthly cycle is called the **menstrual cycle** (from the Latin *mensis* meaning a month). Egg production becomes more and more irregular during the menopause, and stops altogether by the age of about 50.

Figure 9.1 shows how the different events of the menstrual cycle are related. Notice the effects of different hormones. At puberty, each ovary contains about 200 000 immature egg follicles. Each month the pituitary hormones **follicle stimulating hormone** (FSH) and **leutinising hormone** (LH) stimulate the growth of around 20 follicles. One (occasionally more) grows more rapidly than the others. FSH and LH also stimulate the ovaries to produce **oestrogen** hormones which:

- prepare the lining of the uterus (**endometrium**) for implantation of the embryo should the egg be fertilised;
- exert a **negative feedback** effect, reducing FSH release.

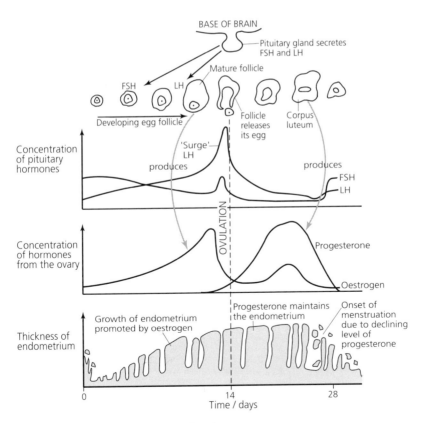

Figure 9.1 Events of the menstrual cycle.

Towards mid-cycle still higher oestrogen levels plus the hormone **progesterone** produced by pre-ovulatory follicles exert a **positive feedback** effect, stimulating the pituitary to release more LH. The surge of LH stimulates the mature follicle to release its egg (**ovulation**). Figure 9.2 shows the interaction of events which lead to ovulation.

The menstrual cycle can affect a woman's emotions. Some women are hardly affected at all, but others feel irritable and below their best just before and during menstruation. A few women experience severe mood swings and physical signs that include changes in appetite. These symptoms are diagnosed as **pre-menstrual syndrome (PMS)**. During the menstrual cycle, the symptoms fluctuate with symptom-free intervals when the woman feels well. The origin of PMS is not clear, but exaggerated fluctuations in oestrogen levels may cause the symptoms directly or change the activity of neurotransmitters in the brain with subsequent knock-on effects.

Following ovulation, the empty follicle is called the **corpus luteum**. It produces the hormone **progesterone** which maintains the endometrium for implantation and inhibits further production of FSH and LH.

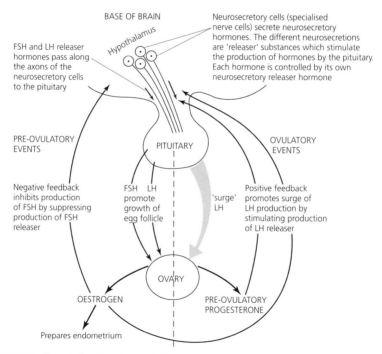

Figure 9.2 Events leading to ovulation.

If the egg is not fertilised, then the corpus luteum breaks down. The subsequent reduction in the amount of progesterone circulating in the blood means the endometrium is no longer maintained. Its thick lining of cells and blood vessels breaks down releasing blood and tissues (**menstruation**). This **menstrual flow** marks the onset of the **period** which lasts for several days. The uterus then returns to its resting state and a new menstrual cycle begins.

If the egg is fertilised, then the developing **placenta** takes over the role of the corpus luteum. It maintains a high level of progesterone in the blood with the result that the endometrium remains intact, providing an environment suitable for the development of the fetus. The high level of progesterone also continues to inhibit the production of FSH and LH, preventing the development of more follicles and release of eggs. Ovulation is therefore prevented during pregnancy and the menstrual cycle stops. When the baby is born, the level of progesterone falls and FSH and LH are released once more, restarting the menstrual cycle.

Menopause and hormone replacement therapy

At around the age of 45 years a woman's ovaries become less sensitive to the effects of FSH and LH. Oestrogen production declines with the result that FSH levels rise (figure 9.2). These fluctuations cause the menstrual disturbances experienced by some women approaching the menopause. As time passes, the woman's periods become less frequent and eventually they stop altogether – a sign that she has reached the menopause.

Some menopausal women experience a 'burning' dryness of the vagina and a feeling of heat centred on the face, neck and chest (hot flushes). These symptoms are due to the low levels of oestrogen, and may be relieved with **hormone replacement therapy (HRT)**. The woman takes small doses of oestrogen either as a daily tablet or as a body patch which slowly releases the hormone through the skin. As well as relieving the symptoms of menopause, in the long term HRT reduces the risk of heart disease and prevents (or at least delays) the development of osteoporosis (page 18).

9.2 Formation and role of the placenta

Fertilisation occurs when the sperm nucleus fuses with the egg nucleus to form a **zygote**. This is the moment of **conception** and the woman is now pregnant. The zygote travels down the Fallopian tube, dividing by **mitosis** as it goes, forming a ball of cells. The journey may take up to seven days, and by the time the ball of cells reaches the uterus it has formed an **embryo**. **Implantation** occurs when the embryo becomes embedded in the endometrium.

Finger-like extensions called **villi** project from the embryo into the endometrium. The surfaces of the embryo and endometrium bind together firmly forming the placenta. During the next few weeks the embryo develops into a fetus attached to the placenta by the **umbilical cord**. Blood vessels running through the umbilical cord connect the blood system of the fetus to the placenta, providing a route for the exchange of food, gases and wastes between mother and fetus. The fetal blood system is not connected to the blood system of the mother directly; the exchange of materials between mother and fetus depends on diffusion across the thin wall of the placenta (figure 9.3).

Passage of drugs across the placenta

All drugs – be they illegal, social or pharmaceutical – pass through the placenta to some extent. Their transfer is more rapid in the later stages of pregnancy as the surface area of the placenta increases in size. Cocaine, heroin and marijuana are examples of illegal drugs. If taken by the mother they may affect development of the fetus. Babies of drug-addicted mothers tend to be smaller than usual, born early and may have congenital abnormalities.

Ethanol (alcohol) is an example of a social drug. It passes across the placenta very easily. A pregnant woman who drinks beer, wine and/or

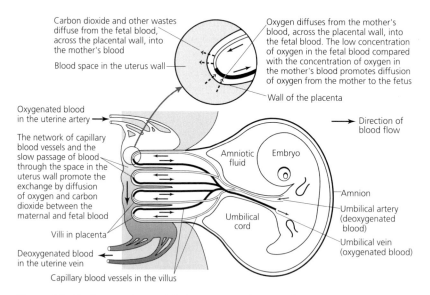

Figure 9.3 Exchange of materials between mother and fetus. Most nutrients cross the placenta from mother to fetus by active transport. Oxygen (from the mother) and carbon dioxide and urea (from the fetus) cross by diffusion. The placenta produces a number of hormones, including oestrogen, progesterone and human chorionic gonadotrophin (page 137).

spirits increases the risk of the fetus developing abnormally. Fetal growth is also reduced. **Fetal alcohol syndrome** may occur if the pregnant woman drinks heavily. At birth the baby is smaller than average, may be mentally retarded and may suffer heart problems. The facial bones may also be incorrectly developed, giving an abnormal look to the face.

Evidence suggests that pregnant women should not smoke. Nicotine (another social drug) and other chemicals in cigarette smoke enter the mother's bloodstream and cross the placenta, increasing the risk of premature birth. Also, babies born to mothers who smoke, on average weigh less than babies born to non-smokers. Reduced blood flow to the placenta prevents the fetus from receiving all of the nutrients it needs from the mother, and higher blood levels of carbon monoxide reduce the uptake of oxygen.

To protect unborn children from the possible harm caused by drugs, advice to pregnant women includes:

- Do not take illegal drugs.
- Do not smoke or drink alcohol.
- Avoid taking pharmaceutical medicines and drugs unless treatment for disease is necessary. **Remember**, all drugs may affect the fetus adversely.

Viral infections

Infections of the mother can have indirect and direct effects on the fetus. Indirect effects may interfere with the physiology of the placenta, altering the exchange of nutrients and respiratory gases. Direct effects depend on the pathogens penetrating the placenta and infecting the fetus. Although viruses are very small and might be expected to cross the placenta with relative ease, most do not affect the fetus unless the mother's infection is severe. However, there are exceptions.

Rubella

Pink spots covering the body, arms, legs and face are symptomatic of German measles, which is caused by the rubella virus. The disease is not serious in an adult. At worst there may be a fever and the lymph glands swell up. However, it is much more serious for a fetus if its mother is infected with rubella during the first four months of pregnancy. Infection of the fetus is almost certain. The virus crosses the placenta and invades actively dividing cells, altering their genetic make-up. Growth of the fetus slows and damage to developing tissues is widespread. In particular, the eye lens (causing cataracts) and ears (causing deafness) may be affected, and the chambers of the heart damaged. Up to 90% of babies whose mothers catch German measles when pregnant are affected. This is why it is important for girls to be vaccinated against the rubella virus before they have children.

Human immunodeficiency virus

Women infected with human immunodeficiency virus (page 6) who become pregnant have a 20–40% chance of transmitting the virus to the fetus. All infected fetuses are antibody positive (page 7) and may go on to develop AIDS. The mother's HIV infection does not adversely affect the progress of the developing fetus, nor does pregnancy adversely affect the progress of HIV infection in the mother.

Pregnant women infected with HIV should be counselled. They are generally given the opportunity to terminate the pregnancy (abortion) rather than risk having a baby infected with HIV.

9.3 Looking after the pregnant woman

The term **antenatal care** covers the advice given and the techniques used to look after the pregnant woman. It aims to ensure that:

- the mother remains healthy during pregnancy;
- complications of pregnancy are detected at an early stage and managed appropriately;
- the fears and anxieties of the mother (and father) are discussed and reassurance given where appropriate;
- the mother knows about the procedures and their outcomes during pregnancy and birth;
- the mother and father know how to look after the baby.

Antenatal care may be given by the mother's doctor (general practitioner), in a clinic run by the nurse or midwife, or in a hospital clinic. The pregnant woman should know what to eat to make sure that she and the developing fetus are properly nourished. Dietary advice for the pregnant woman is discussed in chapter 6.

Screening

Different techniques are used to **screen** the pregnant woman. Screening aims to detect potentially dangerous conditions at an early stage in pregnancy. Measuring the woman's blood pressure during pregnancy is a simple form of screening. Permanently raised blood pressure is a threat to the health of the woman and the developing fetus. More sophisticated techniques aim to screen for genetic defects such as **Down's syndrome**, defects in the development of the central nervous system (e.g. spina bifida) and single gene defects using **DNA probes** (page 119).

Ultrasound scanning

The **ultrasound scanner** produces images which can be used to follow the progress of the developing fetus. The scanner is placed over the mother's abdomen and the images displayed on a TV monitor connected

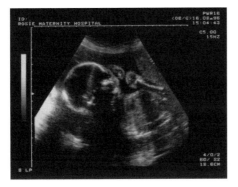

Figure 9.4 Ultrasound scan of fetus.

to the scanner (figure 9.4). The images make it possible to detect the position of the fetus, its size and the presence of more than one fetus. They also help diagnose a variety of fetal defects.

Ultrasound scanning of the pregnant woman has made a considerable impact on antenatal care. The need for X-ray images is much reduced and the information gained helps identify medical problems at different stages in pregnancy as well as reassuring parents that the fetus is healthy.

Amniocentesis

The fetus sheds living cells into the **amniotic fluid**. These cells can be centrifuged, grown in the laboratory and a **karyotype** made which can be examined for genetic defects. Having identified the position of the fetus using ultrasound, a sample of fluid is withdrawn from the amniotic cavity using a thin needle. There is a slight increase in the risk of miscarriage following amniocentesis. Figure 9.5 shows the karyotype of a male fetus. The chromosomes from the nucleus of a body cell have been photographed under the high-power lens of a light microscope. The photograph of the chromosomes has been cut up and the chromosomes arranged into **homologous pairs** (the pairs that form during meiosis) and in order of size.

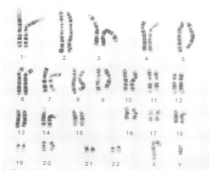

Figure 9.5 Karyotype of a male fetus.

Chorionic villus sampling

In this procedure, a small tube is introduced through the cervix and guided to the edge of the placenta using ultrasound. A small sample of tissue from a villus (page 88) is sucked into the tube. A karyotype is made from the cells of the tissue sample and examined for genetic defects.

Chorionic villus sampling produces results for analysis four to six weeks earlier in pregnancy, but may be associated with a slightly greater risk of miscarriage (1–2%) than amniocentesis (0.5–1%).

Antenatal visits

Most women have a good idea that they are pregnant when they first visit a doctor to confirm the diagnosis. Questions are asked about previous pregnancies (if any), family history and other matters, and the doctor will carry out a physical examination. Samples of blood and urine are taken and sent for routine laboratory testing.

At each antenatal visit, the woman's blood pressure is usually measured. Normally blood pressure remains constant until the last nine weeks of pregnancy when a small increase may occur. Raised blood pressure early in pregnancy may warn of the development of **pregnancy-induced hypertension**. Regular weighing is often thought of as a convenient method for keeping track of fetal growth and for detecting problems. However, careful studies have shown that there is little medical value in measuring a woman's weight during pregnancy.

Most babies are born head first, but sometimes the baby's buttocks or legs lead the way (**breech presentation**). Antenatal visits during the later stages of pregnancy allow the doctor to monitor the position of the fetus relative to the mother's pelvis. Breech births are often quite difficult, and precautions can be taken to prevent damage to the mother and/or baby should a breech birth seem likely.

9.4 Giving birth

To be born, the baby must pass through the birth canal propelled by rhythmic contractions of the uterus. When the contractions start, the events of **labour** begin. **Prostaglandins** and the hormone **oxytocin** play important roles during the onset of labour, but the reason why labour starts is still not clear. It seems that in late pregnancy the number of oxytocin receptors on the muscle cells of the uterus increases. Oxytocin binds to the receptors, promoting the release of prostaglandins which stimulate the uterus to contract. It may also promote the passage of calcium ions (Ca^{2+}) which activate actin and myosin to produce shortening of the muscle fibres. However, hormones are not the whole story. Other factors (structural, nervous, nutritional and circulatory) combine to initiate the events of labour.

Lactogenic hormone (LTH) from the pituitary gland stimulates the tissues of the mammary glands (breasts) to produce milk (lactation). Oestrogen produced by the placenta inhibits the production of LTH during pregnancy. When the placenta is expelled following birth, oestrogen levels fall, removing the inhibition of LTH production. Levels of LTH increase and lactation begins.

9.5 Contraception

If a couple want to have sexual intercourse but do not want to have children they must use some form of **contraception** to prevent pregnancy. Using methods of contraception enables people to choose how many children they want and when to have them. Leaving intervals of two years or more between children is better for a woman's health. Table 9.2 lists different methods of contraception and how they work.

Barrier methods

The **male condom** is a thin-walled sheath, generally made of latex lubricated with silicone and sealed in an aluminium sachet. It is rolled onto the erect penis before intercourse. The penis and condom must be removed from the woman's vagina immediately after ejaculation to avoid any spillage of sperm. Condoms are widely available and give

Table 9.2. Methods of contraception

How the contraceptive works	Method of contraception
Prevents sperm from reaching the egg	Male condom (sheath)
	Female condom
	Spermicides
	Diaphragm and cap

Prevents eggs from being produced	Hormonal contraceptives delivered in the form of:
	    pills
	    injectables
	    implants

Prevents the fertilised egg from developing in the uterus	Intrauterine devices (IUDs)

considerable protection against the transfer of sexually transmitted diseases including HIV.

The **female condom** is a thin-walled sheath made of polyurethane plastic. It is closed at one end and open at the other. A ring at the closed end helps the woman to insert the condom into her vagina before sexual intercourse. A ring at the open end remains outside the body, pushed flat against the labia. The penis is guided into the sheath which lines the vagina. After the penis is removed following ejaculation, the ring at the open end is twisted to make sure no sperm is spilt. The sheath is then gently pulled from the vagina.

Spermicidal creams kill sperm. An applicator is used to put the spermicide inside the vagina just before intercourse. Spermicides are not very effective on their own and are more often used as back-up with other methods.

The **vaginal diaphragm** and **cervical cap** are dome-shaped devices made of plastic or latex attached to a spring rim. The diaphragm comes in different sizes and fits across the vagina. A woman is taught to insert the device by her doctor or at a family planning clinic. It can be inserted each day or just before intercourse, and must remain in place for about six hours afterwards before removal and cleaning. Spermicidal cream smeared around the rim may offer additional protection, and to some extent destroys HIV. The cap is fitted by a doctor. The techniques for insertion and removal are the same as that for the diaphragm.

Hormonal contraceptives

Hormonal contraceptives contain oestrogen and progesterone, or progesterone alone. Oestrogen inhibits FSH secretion and reduces LH secretion, preventing ovulation (figure 9.2). The progesterone inhibits LH secretion further, makes the mucus around the cervix less easy for sperm to penetrate and causes changes in the endometrium of the uterus. Hormonal contraceptives taken as pills are called **oral contraceptives**. There are various formulations:

- The **combined oral contraceptive (COC)** is very effective and chosen by most women in preference to the progesterone-only pill. A small amount of synthetic oestrogen (>50 mg of ethinyl oestradiol) is combined with one of several types of progesterone. The combination is called the 'low-dose pill'.
- The **progesterone-only pill (POP)**, called the 'mini-pill', is suitable for women who are breastfeeding or who may be at risk if they take the COC.

Injectable hormone contraceptives contain synthetic progesterone. Once injected, the hormone is slowly released within the body over two or three months. Injectables are useful for women who find it difficult to take the pill every day or experience problems with other forms of contraception. **Implants** consist of capsules containing synthetic progesterone. The capsules are inserted under the skin of the forearm. As with other progesterone-only formulations such as POPs and injectables, the woman may experience monthly bleeds.

Side effects of combined oral contraceptives (COCs)

The use of COCs gives rise to two main areas of concern: an increased risk of heart disease and some types of cancer. The risk to COC users of blood clot formation is due to an increased concentration of fibrinogen and different clotting factors (page 39). Smoking and obesity increase this risk further. The use of COCs also leads to a small increase in systolic blood pressure (page 46) due to an increased sensitivity to the progesterone and (possibly) oestrogen content of the pill. A woman who uses low-dose COCs reduces the risks, and overall reduces the risk of heart attack (page 39), unless she is a smoker, overweight and more than 35 years old, when a small increased risk occurs. Women in their 30s who have been taking the pill for five years or more before their first pregnancy are also at slightly greater risk of developing breast cancer.

Other possible side effects occurring in women using COCs include:

- weight gain;
- nausea and vomiting;
- headaches and migraine;
- vaginal discharge.

These effects are often temporary and settle down once the body has adjusted to the changed hormonal environment. However, concern about heart disease and the cancers mentioned above means that women with a history of heart disease or hypertension, or who have an oestrogen-dependent cancer, should not choose COCs as their method of contraception.

Intrauterine devices

Intrauterine devices (IUDs) are fitted inside the uterus by a doctor. The IUD touches the inner wall of the uterus and prevents implantation of the embryo. The IUD can be removed by a doctor by pulling on the strings attached to it which pass through the cervix. There are several types of IUD. In one type, fine copper wire surrounds the stem. The copper prevents sperm from fertilising the egg. The stem of another type contains synthetic progesterone. The device works in the same way as the progesterone-only pill.

During insertion of the IUD, there is a risk of perforating the wall of the uterus. However, the risk is slight and depends on the skill of the doctor performing the insertion. Muscular contractions of the uterus may also expel the IUD, especially during a period. Nevertheless, once inserted and providing there are no complications, the IUD prevents pregnancy very effectively for up to seven years.

Natural methods

All of the methods of contraception in table 9.2 depend on chemicals or a mechanical device to be effective. The **rhythm method** uses none of these, but depends on the woman (and possibly her partner) understanding how her menstrual cycle works. During the menstrual cycle, intercourse is most likely to lead to pregnancy at the time when ovulation occurs. Figure 9.6 shows the sorts of changes in a woman's body temperature that occur during her menstrual cycle. A slight increase in body temperature is a signal that she has ovulated, and that she should not have intercourse until her temperature drops to its pre-ovulation value. Unfortunately, the menstrual cycle is not always predictable. The cycle can vary a good deal, especially in teenagers, which makes it difficult to predict whether or not it is safe to have intercourse. However, the rhythm method is a natural form of contraception, and it is used mostly by people whose religion does not permit other methods.

The **periodic abstinence method** depends on the woman detecting the type of mucus at the entrance to the vagina each morning. At around the time of ovulation, the appearance, quantity and consistency of the mucus changes. The nature of the mucus signals when the woman should not have intercourse. The co-operation of the woman's partner is essential if pregnancy is to be avoided.

Sterilisation

Sterilisation involves a minor operation. In a man, the sperm ducts are tied off and cut by the surgeon. The man can still ejaculate as the ducts are cut below the seminal vesicles which produce seminal fluid, but his

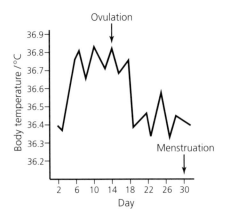

Figure 9.6 Changes in body temperature during the menstrual cycle.

semen will not contain any sperm. In a woman, the oviducts are tied off and cut. This prevents the sperm from reaching the egg. Although some sterilisation operations can be reversed, this is not usually the case, so a man or woman who is sterilised has to be very sure that he or she no longer wants children.

The **Pearl Index** quantifies the effectiveness of the various methods of contraception. It calculates the unintended pregnancy rate from the formula:

$$\frac{\text{number of unintended pregnancies}}{\text{total months of exposure to pregnancy}} \times 1200$$

The result gives a failure rate per 100 woman years. Table 9.3 compares the reliability of different methods of contraception.

Table 9.3. The reliability of contraceptive methods

Method	Reliability
No method	Very unreliable
Rhythm method	Unreliable without expert help
Diaphragm with spermicide	Quite reliable when fitted well
Sheath	Quite reliable if used properly
IUDs	Reliable
The pill	Very reliable

9.6 Abortion

The time during which the fetus develops inside the mother's uterus is called the **gestation period**. It normally lasts for around 38 weeks. However, the fetus is **viable** (capable of surviving independently) when the gestation period has reached 22 weeks or more. **Abortion** is defined by the World Health Organisation as 'removal of a fetus from the uterus before it is viable'. If the removal is natural (**spontaneous**) then many doctors describe the event as a **miscarriage**. The term abortion is usually confined to the deliberate (**induced**) removal of the fetus.

In the early weeks of pregnancy (0–10 weeks), 70% of the miscarriages occur because of defects in the fertilised egg or because the fetus is not developing normally. Chromosomal abnormalities are a common underlying cause of early miscarriage. After 10 weeks of pregnancy, factors concerning the mother become more common. For example, infections and abnormalities of the uterus may cause the fetus to detach from the placenta. As the placental function fails, the uterus begins to contract and miscarriage occurs.

In many countries, legalised abortion protects women from the dangers of 'backstreet' abortions. Before legislation, illegal abortions were often performed in unhygienic conditions and carried a high risk of disease and even death. Today, an abortion performed by medical staff in a well-equipped clinic is followed by few complications, especially when undertaken in the first 12 weeks of pregnancy.

Most abortions are performed for social reasons or because the pregnant woman feels psychologically unprepared for a baby. In about 5% of cases there are medical reasons for abortion. For example, abortion might be advisable for a woman suffering from severe heart or kidney failure, or if serious genetic defects in the fetus are detected. Most women think very hard about the implications of having an abortion before taking the decision to have one. For many it is a difficult time and support from family, friends and trained counsellors is often needed.

Methods of abortion

Abortion is safest between the 6th and 12th weeks of pregnancy. It may be induced by surgical or medical methods:

- *Surgical methods* – the contents of the uterus are sucked out using a device called a **suction curette**. The woman is given a local or general anaesthetic. Bleeding from the uterus occurs for about six days following the operation. A course of antibiotics (page 15) is often prescribed to prevent infection.
- *Medical methods* – the woman is prescribed **mifepristone** which is a progesterone antagonist (see page 112 for the role of progesterone during pregnancy), followed 36–48 hours later by prostaglandin inserted as a pessary (soluble capsule) into the vagina every six hours for four doses. The prostaglandin promotes contraction of the uterus. If abortion does not begin within 24 hours, then four more pessaries are inserted at three-hourly intervals. In most cases abortion then begins. There may be severe discomfort and most women need pain relief. Bleeding from the uterus persists for about nine days, and some women feel sick.

Abortions carried out after the 12th week of pregnancy may involve the use of **sponge forceps** and suction to remove the fetus and placenta. Alternatively, the combination of mifepristone and prostaglandin may be used, but suction is sometimes needed to remove remnants of the placenta and fetal tissue.

Amniocentisis, chorionic villus sampling and other antenatal screening techniques (page 90) allow potentially harmful genetic conditions to be detected in developing fetuses. The information may help expectant parents who have reason to be worried about the possibility of genetic disorders. **Genetic counselling** may help couples decide whether to continue with a pregnancy when they know their baby has a genetic disorder. However, the decision is rarely simple. Examples of circumstances that some people have to deal with are listed below. Think about them carefully. Also remember that no screening procedure can be relied upon to be 100% accurate.

Following screening a pregnant woman has been told that her child will be born with one of the following genetic disorders:

- Down's syndrome;
- a genetic disease from which the child will die within twelve months of birth;
- a genetic disease which will cause gradual deterioration in health – the child will probably die between the ages of 20 and 30.

What are the choices? Should abortion be chosen in some of these circumstances? Should the woman choose to give birth to her baby, and then seek the best medical advice for the problems the baby has inherited? This series of questions highlights the problems of choice and decision of action.

Continuous ill health causes enormous strain in a family and may even make other people ill with the worry and extra work of constant care. Where does the balance of concern lie? Various religions deal with difficult moral issues. Are they a guide for the decisions to be made? Do we know how people who are very ill feel about their lives? We may think that their lives do not seem worthwhile, but they may be very happy within themselves. Who is to judge? Remember, too, that diseases today that are untreatable may, with scientific progress, be curable tomorrow. Yet more and more questions! They show how difficult it is to come to hard and fast conclusions.

Amniocentesis and ultrasound can be used to identify the sex of a fetus at an early stage in pregnancy. In some countries, sons are valued more highly than daughters. So where procedures to determine the sex of a fetus are readily available, female fetuses are aborted in large numbers. Abortion therefore can be a method of family planning – in these cases in favour of males rather than females.

However you approach the questions raised above, it is difficult to judge the answers. There are no easy solutions.

9.7 Infertility

Couples are usually thought to be infertile if they have regular, unprotected intercourse for 12 months without pregnancy occurring. About 10% of couples are infertile. Of these, about 40% of cases are due to male infertility, 35% are due to female infertility and 25% have unknown causes.

Male infertility

Normal semen contains more than 20 million sperm per ml, more than 50% of which are healthy in appearance and mobility. A man's fertility is affected if the sperm count falls below 20 million per ml (**oligospermia**). Table 9.4 lists the various categories of male infertility. In cases of severe and absolute infertility, a blood sample is taken to measure the man's FSH levels. Raised levels of FSH suggest malfunction of the testes.

Pregnancy is unusual in cases where the man is severely infertile, and impossible when infertility is absolute. One remedy is insemination of the woman with semen from another man (donor). Should couples choose this option, the woman is artificially inseminated with donor semen each month, for up to 12 months if necessary. Over 65% of women who choose donor insemination become pregnant.

In cases of relative infertility, attempts have been made to improve the sperm count using tablets of **testosterone** (the male hormone which promotes sperm formation). However, the treatment does not seem to improve the pregnancy rate, compared with that of couples where the man who is relatively infertile is untreated and where the couple persist in unprotected sex. Relative infertility is more successfully treated using *in vitro* fertilisation (see below).

Female infertility

A variety of factors affect fertility in women:
- damage to the Fallopian tubes prevents the passage of sperm;
- sperm in the vagina cannot penetrate the mucus around the cervix en route for the uterus;
- ovulation either does not occur or occurs only infrequently;

Table 9.4. Male infertility

Category	Sperm count/per ml
Relative infertility	< 20 million
Severe infertility	< 5 million
Absolute infertility	0

- abnormalities of the uterus, e.g. failure of the pre-embryo to implant.

Measurement of progesterone levels in the blood mid-way through the second half of the menstrual cycle (page 85) is the most effective way of finding out if a woman is ovulating normally. Depressed levels indicate a failure to ovulate. Treatment aims to stimulate ovulation. Tablets of the anti-oestrogen drug **clomiphene** make tissues insensitive to oestrogen by binding onto oestrogen receptors in target cells. The negative feedback control by oestrogen on the pituitary is inhibited (page 85) with the result that FSH and LH levels increase. Ovulation is induced in up to 80% of women treated with clomiphene.

The methods used to detect blockage of the Fallopian tubes depend on tracking dyes (or other liquids that can be imaged) as they pass through the uterus and Fallopian tubes. Once the blockage is identified, treatment aims to clear the tubes so that sperm can pass through and meet the egg.

Failure of sperm to penetrate the cervical mucus at the time of ovulation is more likely to be due to defective sperm function than other causes. Sperm–cervical mucus tests aim to identify the particular problem so that appropriate treatment can be offered.

In vitro **fertilisation (IVF)** techniques have given new hope for infertile couples. Hormonal treatment induces ovulation and the eggs are then retrieved from the woman and prepared for fertilisation. Sperm are added to selected eggs, and two or three fertilised eggs are then transferred into the uterus. Repeated IVF results in around 40% of treated women giving birth to a healthy baby.

Are environmental pollutants altering the reproductive health of humans? A vast number of industrial and agricultural chemicals are thought to mimic or interfere with sex hormones. Such compounds include products of petrol combustion such as polycrylic aromatic hydrocarbons, phthalates (which are ingredients in paints, inks and adhesives, and added as plasticisers in plastics), polychlorinated biphenyls (PCBs) and insecticides such as DDT, dieldrin and aldrin. However, the evidence is far from clear. For example, claims that PCBs and DDT act like oestrogen result from work linking them with egg infertility in different bird species. Some scientists suggest that oestrogen mimics in the environment are contributing to the increase in the rate of breast cancer. However, recent reports indicate that there has been no increase in deaths from breast cancer since the chemicals were introduced. Who is right? It is very difficult to unravel cause and effect. Some people think absolute proof is not possible, but that on the basis of the evidence so far we should reduce the release of potentially harmful substances as a safeguard against any possible future problems.

The brain: memory, ageing and the effects of drugs

The title of this chapter raises questions that are at the leading edge of research. To make sense of this subject, we can investigate brain structure, its neurones (nerve cells) and synapses or its biochemistry, or seek a route for our understanding through functional deficiences such as **Alzheimer's disease, Creutzfeldt-Jacob disease** that constitute brain **dementia**. In fact, the whole picture only emerges through the combination of level upon level of organisation – molecules to memory. We shall adopt just such a multilevel approach to glimpse the functioning brain at work in health and disease.

The human brain weighs about 1.3 kg. Divided into different regions – forebrain, midbrain and hindbrain – it is the body's thinking and control centre. Reactions to stimuli that are under the brain's control are called **voluntary** responses. Memory and learning are also controlled by the brain.

The **neurones** in the brain are called **multipolar** neurones because each one has numerous **dendrites** which can form **synapses** with incoming **axons**, connecting each multipolar neurone to as many as 80 000 other neurones. It has been estimated that the human brain consists of up to 20 000 million neurones, but this does not take into account the non-neural **glia** cells in which neurones are embedded. Supporting, nurturing and protecting the neurones, glia cells outnumber neurones ten-fold.

10.1 Memory

Today, understanding the mechanisms of memory is one of the great scientific challenges. Memory allows us to recall past experiences, connecting learning to remembering. If the functions of the brain are to be explained within the context of the structures which form the brain, and since learning and memory are components of brain function, then learning and memory must bring about changes in brain structures. Will your brain change, therefore, as a result of reading and remembering this book? If there are changes, will they leave a memory trace of your activity? Evidence from research on humans and other animals suggests that memory formation does indeed leave structural, physiological and biochemical traces (sometimes called an **engram**) which can be investigated, analysed and interpreted within the context of the experiences remembered.

A memory of an event is built up over a period of hours after the event has occurred. Initially, short-term changes take place in the electrical properties and responsiveness of sets of neurones 'coding' for the memory. These then give way to biochemical processes such as the reconstruction and formation of new synapses which represent the memory permanently in another set of neurones. Evidence from human studies suggests that this process results in **short-term memory** and **long-term memory**, and that a region of the brain called the **hippocampus** is involved in the transition between the two.

However, distinguishing memory as short-term or long-term is too simplistic. Attempts to describe and classify the main features of memory show that in reality it is more complex. For example, as a result of brain damage some people can remember *how* to ride a bicycle but forget *that* the machine is called a bicycle. Remembering *how* and knowing *that* seem to be different processes and are classified accordingly. *How* memory is called **procedural** skill or habit memory. *That* memory is called **declarative**. Furthermore, procedural memory does not seem to involve short- and long-term memory processes. **Associative** memory acquires facts and figures and holds them in long-term storage. **Working** memory complements associative memory by activating and storing symbolic information in the short term. Constructing this sentence and planning chess moves, for example, involve the use of working memory. Working memory is fundamental to language, to learning and to reason.

Recognising different forms of memory raises important questions. Are different parts of the brain responsible for different types of memory, or are the functions of the brain integrated? Do changes in brain structure, physiology and biochemistry associated with memory formation differ depending on the type of memory stored? These are some of the topics of current research.

Structural basis of memory

The human brain is dominated by the cerebral hemispheres whose surfaces are covered by the **cerebral cortex**. Wrinkling and folding increase the surface area of the cortex and hence its capacity for complex activity. In the 1950s, activities controlled by the cortex were mapped using electrodes as probes through which a current was passed to electrically stimulate the cells in different areas of the cortex. Patients reported a range of responses, including memories of past experiences, depending on the area stimulated. Memory recall and visual flashbacks seemed to be particularly localised in the **temporal lobe**. However, the investigations prompted new questions. Were the memories real or imagined? Did stimulation unlock memories stored in the region that was stimulated, or was there communication with other regions where they were stored?

> The brain is insensitive to pain. This means that during surgical operations which expose the brain, patients need only a local anaesthetic and are therefore able to report the effects of stimulating different areas of the cortex using electrodes.

Subsequent research has revealed the main regions of the brain thought to be involved in the formation and storage of memory (figure 10.1). Current work suggests that the different regions form an interconnected network of neuronal pathways. Long-term memory is established when information generated by sensory inputs traverses all of the pathways.

Physiological basis of memory

Although tracing neuronal pathways through the brain identifies routes through which information flows to establish memories, 'what makes memory?' remains an open question. Possible answers are coming from

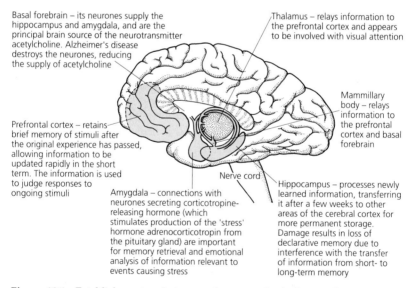

Basal forebrain – its neurones supply the hippocampus and amygdala, and are the principal brain source of the neurotransmitter acetylcholine. Alzheimer's disease destroys the neurones, reducing the supply of acetylcholine

Thalamus – relays information to the prefrontal cortex and appears to be involved with visual attention

Mammillary body – relays information to the prefrontal cortex and basal forebrain

Prefrontal cortex – retains brief memory of stimuli after the original experience has passed, allowing information to be updated rapidly in the short term. The information is used to judge responses to ongoing stimuli

Nerve cord

Amygdala – connections with neurones secreting corticotropine-releasing hormone (which stimulates production of the 'stress' hormone adrenocorticotropin from the pituitary gland) are important for memory retrieval and emotional analysis of information relevant to events causing stress

Hippocampus – processes newly learned information, transferring it after a few weeks to other areas of the cerebral cortex for more permanent storage. Damage results in loss of declarative memory due to interference with the transfer of information from short- to long-term memory

Figure 10.1 Establishment and storage of memory in the human brain. Loss of memory results from damage to any of the structures shown. The type of memory loss depends on which structures are damaged. For example, Korsakoff's syndrome develops in chronic alcoholics due to thiamine deficiency. The thalamus and mammillary body degenerate causing memory loss of recent events. Sufferers are unable to carry out verbal or non-verbal memory tasks, remember simple facts or plan straightforward jobs.

work on changes that occur at cellular and molecular levels when animals learn and remember new activities.

Different models to explain how cellular mechanisms form memories have been put forward since the beginning of the twentieth century. Two of the more recent models for which there is evidence from learning and memory studies in different animals are shown in figure 10.2. The events of model A occur in the hippocampus (figure 10.1) where they are responsible for synaptic changes that are important for spatial memory (e.g. the ability to remember the way home through a maze of streets). Model B events seem to contribute to associative memory (see overleaf).

Figure 10.2 poses two questions: what is meant by 'strengthening synaptic connections, and what is the significance of the strengthening? In the 1960s different experiments showed that when different regions of the cortex were electrically stimulated, there were long-lasting increases in the spontaneous electrical activity of these regions. In 1973, attention focused on the hippocampus and the neural pathways feeding it. In an important experiment using anaesthetised rabbits, stimulating electrodes were placed on one of the nerves leading to the hippocampus and recording electrodes were located within the hippocampus itself. Brief (10 seconds) high frequency stimulation of the incoming nerve produced an increase in synaptic strength and in lasting increase (10 hours) in the firing of the hippocampal neurones. The event was called **long-term potentiation (LTP)**. Non-anaesthetised animals implanted with permanent electrodes showed LTP lasting 16 weeks after stimulation.

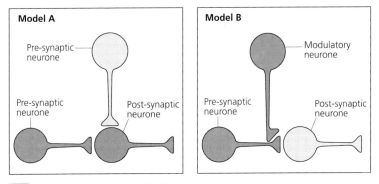

■ Indicates simultaneous activity in neurones

Figure 10.2 Strengthening synaptic connections. Simultaneous activity in the pre-synaptic and post-synaptic neurones strengthens the synaptic connections between them (model A). In model B, the synaptic connections can be strengthened by simultaneous activity in the pre-synaptic and modulatory neurones, without activity in the post-synaptic neurone. Although only single synapses are shown in the models, in reality the processes probably involve hundreds of neurones, each making many thousands of synapses. Learning and remembering even simple tasks is therefore likely to involve whole groups of neurones. (Adapted from Freeman W.H. 1993, Mind and brain, *Scientific American.)*

LTP strengthens synaptic connections, but what is its significance? By the 1970s the hippocampus was known to be involved with memory. So, is LTP the mechanism by which memories are formed? The evidence shows that a lasting change in output (LTP) occurs as a result of a defined input (the initial brief stimulation). Furthermore, for LTP to occur, pre-synaptic and post-synaptic neurones must be active simultaneously (see model A, figure 10.2) with the result that the LTP is specific. In other words, the LTP is restricted in its action to the pathway through which flows information about the experience to be remembered.

Think about the rabbit experiment described above and the sequence of events. LTP appears to proceed in two phases: a brief initial stimulus (the 10 second burst of high frequency stimulation) followed by a longer term maintenance phase (the 10 hours – or 16 weeks in alert animals – of enhanced firing of hippocampal neurones). Are these phases the physiological representation of short-term experience and transfer of the experience to long-term memory?

Evidence from another set of experiments shows that although a weak stimulus cannot initiate LTP on its own, it can do so if it is combined with a strong stimulus from another neuronal pathway (see model B, figure 10.2). In other words, the two inputs (weak and strong) *associate* to produce an effect called **associative LTP**, in the same way as conditioned and unconditioned stimuli must combine for **associative learning** to occur.

Associative learning and memory

This phenomenon was first described by the Russian physiologist Ivan Pavlov (1849–1936). He observed that when food (the **unconditioned stimulus**) was placed in a dog's mouth, the flow of saliva increased. He also observed that the flow of saliva increased as soon as the dog smelt his hand (the **conditioned stimulus**), even before food was placed in its mouth. After a period of presenting the dog with both the personal smell and the taste of food, personal smell alone was enough to make the dog produce as much saliva as if it were given food. In other words, the dog learnt to *associate* a conditioned stimulus (Pavlov's personal smell), which normally would not cause salivation, with the unconditioned stimulus (food) which did cause salivation, so that after the food was withdrawn the conditioned stimulus alone was remembered and produced a response. Does model B, figure 10.2, suggest the physiological basis for associative learning and memory?

We know that the hippocampus is involved in various forms of memory, and that associative LTP occurs there. Is this evidence for the mechanism by which memory is stored, if not for memory itself? There are no apologies for yet another question mark. The chapter begins with questions and promises only a glimpse of the functioning brain at work. Continuing research will provide answers, and doubtless raise yet more questions.

Biochemical basis of memory

Why is simultaneous firing of pre-synaptic and post-synaptic neurones necessary for LTP? Figure 10.3 provides some of the answers. The cascade of biochemical events and interactions between the pre-synaptic and post-synaptic terminals initiate and maintain LTP.

- *Initiating LTP* – depolarisation of the post-synaptic neurone leads to an influx of calcium ions (Ca^{2+}) and activation of different messenger molecules.

- *Synaptic feedback* – the calcium-activated messenger molecules in the post-synaptic neurone promote the release of nitric oxide which diffuses to the pre-synaptic terminal. Here it activates other messenger molecules which promote the release of **neurotransmitter**.

- *Maintaining LTP* – increased release of neurotransmitter from the pre-synaptic neurone continues to depolarise the post-synaptic neurone.

The nitric oxide 'loop' between the post-synaptic and pre-synaptic terminals is an example of positive feedback (page 86) and maintains LTP.

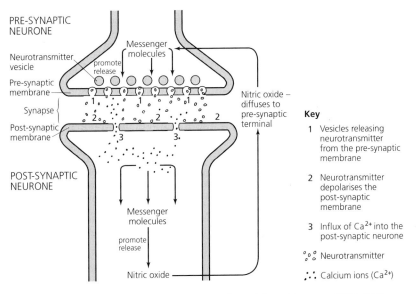

Figure 10.3 Biochemistry of the synapse. (Adapted from Freeman W.H. 1993, Mind and brain, *Scientific American*.)

Inhibiting the synthesis of nitric oxide in the post-snaptic neurone, or absorbing nitric oxide in the synaptic cleft, *blocks* the development of LTP. On the other hand, applying nitric oxide to the synaptic cleft *promotes* the release of neurotransmitter from the pre-synaptic neurone and enhances LTP.

Notice parallels between the biochemical events across the synapse, associative learning and memory and the mechanism of associative LTP. *Conditioned* and *unconditioned* stimuli combine to produce associative learning and memory (page 106); *weak* and *strong* stimuli combine to produce associative LTP – and events across the synapse? Figure 10.3 shows the mechanisms responsible for LTP:

- activation of receptors in the post-synaptic neurone produces nitric oxide;
- nitric oxide promotes transmitter release from the pre-synaptic neurone.

Nitric oxide and neurotransmitter are two independent but associated signals such as those from conditioned and unconditioned stimuli. Their combination ensures that pre-synaptic and post-synaptic neurones are active simultaneously, accounting for the specificity of LTP (page 106).

Storing memory

Associative LTP occurs in the hippocampus, which we know to be important for memory storage. When receptors in the hippocampus are blocked, experimental animals fail to learn simple tasks. So once more we ask the question: is LTP part of the process that stores memories?

Short-term storage (lasting minutes to hours) involves changes in the strength of synaptic connections by means of the physiological and biochemical mechanisms described above. Long-term storage also requires gene activation which promotes the synthesis of proteins necessary for the growth of new synaptic connections. Recent research shows that stimuli of the sort that produce long-term memory lead to an increase in the number of pre-synaptic terminals, and that LTP produces similar changes in the hippocampus.

New learning situations, therefore, continuously modify the brain as memories of the experiences are stored. For example, when a monkey was encouraged to repeatedly touch a revolving disc with the middle three fingers of its hand, it showed expansion of the region of the cortex which controlled the active fingers. Is this why practice improves our ability to play a musical instrument? The neural pathways in the cortex that control finger movement are constantly modified and updated through associated activities, such as playing notes in sequence correctly. Practice, which is the stimulus for the mechanisms that generate LTP, makes for improvement. The result: music is learnt and remembered.

10.2 The ageing brain

For me, Latin at school was a mystery. Fortunately my teenage memory was virtually photographic and learning 600 lines of Virgil's *Aeneid*, although difficult, was not a problem. My Latin master's majestic translation began: 'I sing of arms and of a man... (Arma virumque cano...)', and so the lines rolled on to good effect as, with some success, I jumped the hurdles of first public exams *en route* to Biology. Older and greyer, I now find it difficult to recall yesterday's supper, although fragments of Virgil remain lodged in the recesses of my memory.

The word **eidetic** (from a Greek word meaning 'image') is the technical term for photographic memory, and around 50% of young children seem to have it. Yet eidetic memory is rare in adults. In other words, the reality of memory changes as we grow older. Even so, the changes are not uniform. The way you remember yourself, and the way I remember myself, five years ago are different. For me it seems like yesterday, for you possibly a lifetime! Memory itself is a developmental process, and what you remember over a five-year period represents a change in the quality of memory. For an older person like myself, the memory is stable.

The brain is bombarded with the stimuli of everyday events. As we grow older, information to be memorized is increasingly selected from the barrage of sensory 'noise' around us. This mechanism of **perceptual filtering** ensures that the brain is not 'clogged' with information and registers only those details which are personally significant. As I write, the sound of traffic, distant music and background voices are heard but do not disturb me, because I am not concentrating on them. The incoming information is entering my brain but filtering is unconsciously sorting it according to importance and rejecting most of it. Of course, what is insignificant for me may be significant for someone else. We learn the criteria by which to filter stimuli during our own development. In other words, filtering is an important aspect of our learning to concentrate on information important to us as individuals.

The eidetic memory of childhood does not filter stimuli. All are equally important. The child, therefore, can analyse a wide range of inputs and learn to select key features – helped perhaps by parents and teachers who could be thought of as surrogate filters! These experiences from childhood mould our adult interests and preoccupations.

The weight of the brain declines with age, probably through shrinkage and loss of neurones. Different studies also show a decline in the activity of particular enzymes and other neurochemicals. However, such reductions appear to have little effect on thinking. For example, **positron emission tomographic (PET)** imaging indicates that the brains of healthy people in their eighties are almost as efficient as those of people in their twenties. Also, tests of memory, perception and language in the young and elderly who are healthy show few differences in performance.

Mental processes, however, do seem to change with ageing. The speed of processing seems to slow down, but youthful quickness gives way to more efficient strategies for coping with and manipulating information – in other words, wisdom comes with age! In older people, filtering processes either block out trivial events, or if such items are lodged in the memory they are not recalled. Either way, the brain accumulates, refines and retrieves memories essential to the problems of day-to-day living. These are the processes of **experience**.

Dementia

The term 'dementia' covers a variety of diseases causing loss of memory and reason in the elderly. Until the 1970s, many causes of dementia were thought to be an inevitable part of the ageing process. However, different studies show that only around 5% of people aged between 65 and 75 years show signs of dementia. Although the figure rises in people older than this, the majority in their eighties and nineties can expect to remain symptom-free.

Where dementia does occur, Alzheimer's disease is a leading cause. Figure 10.4 shows the structural abnormalities associated with Alzheimer's disease:

- **Neurofibrillary tangles** of a protein called **tau** accumulate within the cell bodies of neurones. The tangles are insoluble in

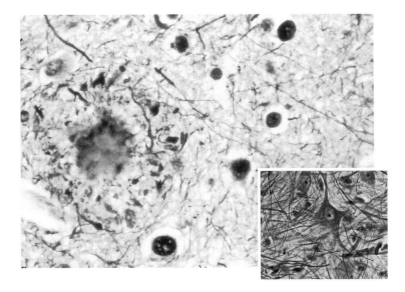

Figure 10.4 Section of brain tissue of an Alzheimer's victim, compared with healthy brain tissue (*inset*). The neurofibrillary tangles and neuritic plaques contain high concentrations of aluminium. Whether or not aluminium causes tangles, or the tangles accumulate aluminium, is unknown.

water and resist enzymatic breakdown. They remain long after the neurones have died.

- **Neuritic plaques,** which are an accumulation of a protein called **amyloid** and degenerating axons. Amyloid protein also accumulates next to and within the walls of blood vessels.

These abnormalities are found in different regions of the cerebral cortex, especially in the hippocampus, amygdala and basal forebrain (figure 10.1). Research shows that the build-up of amyloid protein with the formation of neurofibrillary tangles disrupts the neural pathways serving memory and thinking.

Normal tau protein helps maintain the shape of neurones, but in patients with Alzheimer's it is converted to an abnormal form. The tangles characteristic of Alzheimer's consist of abnormal tau. The number of tangles is proportional to the severity of the patient's dementia. Abnormal tau binds strongly to normal tau, converting it to the abnormal form. Tangles appear as more and more abnormal tau accumulate. Research shows that the proportion of normal tau declines from 97% in normal people to 17% in patients with severe Alzheimer's. Why tau converts from normal to abnormal form is not known, but the search is on for the mechanism that triggers the change.

The role of amyloid protein in Alzheimer's is uncertain. It may directly damage surrounding neurones once a critical concentration is reached, or accumulate and attract other substances that do the damage.

Amyloid protein consists of 42 amino acids. The gene coding for it is located on chromosome 21. Mutations of the gene accelerate deposition of amyloid protein. Down's syndrome (page 118) is caused by an extra copy of chromosome 21 and, perhaps significantly, many people with Down's syndrome eventually develop Alzheimer's. Environmental factors may also play a part. For example, after the Second World War the people living on the Pacific Island of Guam experienced an outbreak of neurological disorders, including an Alzheimer's-like disease. More than 20% of the population died. The problem seems to have originated during the war. Research suggests that the outbreak was triggered by islanders consuming an unusual amino acid found in high concentrations in cycads – a type of gymnosperm which grows locally. Food was prepared from cycad seeds because of shortages of other food. Cycad seeds were no longer a major source of food after the war ended, and the incidence of neurological diseases has dropped dramatically since the 1950s.

Continuing research aims to find answers to the many questions that remain. How do mutations of the amyloid gene accelerate deposition of amyloid protein? Different tissues make amyloid, but why does it accumulate only in the brain? Why are neurones of the hippocampus more sensitive to amyloid than other brain neurones? How can we prevent the destructive processes of Alzheimer's disease? These problems are becoming increasingly urgent as the developed nations face a surge in the numbers of elderly people.

10.3 Effects of drugs

Many drugs have their effects by acting on the protein receptor molecules located in the cell membrane of neurones. Their action promotes or reduces synaptic transmission.

Receptors normally respond to neurotransmitters such as acetylcholine. The response generates nerve impulses in the affected neurone. **Agonists** are drugs that combine with and activate receptors, producing a response. Their action triggers a cascade of physiological and biochemical processes that generate nerve impulses. **Antagonists** are drugs that combine with but do not activate receptors, and therefore do not produce a response. They reduce the probability of neurotransmitters (or other agonists) combining with receptors and therefore block the generation of nerve impulses.

The interaction between a drug and receptor is rather like a lock and key, and depends on how closely the two molecules fit one another. The closer the fit, the more the molecules bind together, and the higher the **affinity** of the drug for the receptor. The **specificity** of a drug is its ability to combine with a particular receptor. Most drugs are relatively selective for a particular type of receptor, binding with that type but not with others. This means that drugs have particular effects which are useful for different treatments. However, specificity is not absolute, and most drugs have unwanted side effects that may or may not be serious. For example, atropine blocks acetylcholine receptors which are found in the eye, intestine, skin, and brain. Its unwanted side effects include blurred vision, dry mouth and constipation. As well as these, though, it has beneficial effects in anaesthesia, the treatment of Parkinson's disease and different complaints of the intestine.

Opiates

Opiates are drugs produced from the opium poppy *Papaver somniferum*. Raw opium is a gum which comes from the dried juice of the seed head of the flower. It is a mixture of many substances including a number of **alkaloids**, which are organic ring compounds containing nitrogen. Two of them (**morphine** and **codeine**) are powerful painkillers (**analgesics**), and another (**papaverine**) is a smooth muscle relaxant. Opium also produces a sense of well-being (euphoria), is highly addictive and often **abused** – a term used to describe the non-medical use of drugs.

Heroin is a semi-synthetic opiate derived from morphine. It is widely abused, producing euphoria and reducing sensitivity to pain. In its pure form, heroin is a white powder which may be smoked ('chasing the dragon') or made up in solution and injected into a vein ('mainlining').

To begin with, people take heroin for the euphoria it induces, but physiological dependence develops rapidly. Addicts continue to use the drug, not so much for its euphoric effect but to avoid the symptoms that follow ('cold turkey'). These vary but are generally unpleasant. Another opiate called **methadone** is often used to treat heroin addicts. Substituted for heroin, withdrawal from methadone is less intense. The dose of methadone is 'tapered off' as the person slowly responds to treatment.

Mode of action

The central nervous system and other tissues in the body produce a class of natural opiates called **endorphins**. Stimulated pain receptors relay pain information through neural pathways in the spinal cord to the brain cortex which registers the stimuli. Endorphins released in response to the painful stimuli bind to endorphin receptors on post-synaptic neurones. The receptors are widely distributed throughout the spinal cord and brain. The endorphin/receptor interaction reduces the production of nerve impulses in the relay pathways and brain, and therefore reduces the pain. Heroin and other opiate drugs are similar in structure to endorphins and also bind to endorphin receptors, especially those concentrated in the brain. The drug/receptor interaction mimics the natural events which reduce pain.

Enkephalins are a group of endorphins which play a role in the integration of sensory information associated with pain and emotional behaviour. Opiate drugs bind to enkephalin receptors concentrated in the **amygdala** of the brain (figure 10.1) – the region particularly associated with feelings of pleasure. The drug/receptor interaction may account for the euphoric effect of opiates. The drug **naxalone** is a specific antagonist of opiate receptors. It blocks the receptor completely and is used in the emergency treatment of opiate drug **overdose**.

The mechanisms underlying opioid dependence are poorly understood. One idea supposes that long-term opiate abuse reduces the normal production of endorphins. The body comes to depend more and more on the drug with the result that addiction develops.

Cocaine

Cocaine is a white powder made from the leaves of the S. American coca shrub. Medically, it is used as a **local anaesthetic**, but its effects on the central nervous system also make it a popular drug of abuse. The drug, also called 'snow', 'coke' and 'C', may be sniffed ('snorting'), injected or smoked. 'Crack' is a highly addictive form of cocaine which is smoked.

Cocaine increases confidence and personal energy, and is also an antidepressant. However, the drug's main danger is the development of a strong psychological dependency.

Mode of action

Cocaine enters the axon through the axon membrane. Once inside, it blocks sodium channels in the axon membrane. The higher the dose the more sodium channels are blocked, until eventually the number of active open channels falls below the minimum necessary to generate a nerve impulse. Nerve block occurs and anaesthesia results. Medically, cocaine is mainly used for the local anaesthesia of body surfaces where its ability to restrict blood vessels (**vasorestriction**) is also useful. For example, **amethocaine** drops are used to anaesthetise the cornea of the eye.

Cocaine also mimics the action of the neurotransmitter noradrenaline. It continuously activates receptors, triggering nerve impulses. There is an intense stimulant effect on the central nervous system and the person experiences a 'high'. Cocaine can have serious psychological effects. Repeated use may produce a state similar to an attack of **schizophrenia**.

Atropine

Deadly nightshade (*Atropa belladonna*) is a source of **atropine**. Medically, it is used to reduce spontaneous contractions of the intestine, and to control heart rate and reduce secretions in the airways during anaesthesia.

Mode of action

Atropine inhibits the effects of acetylcholine by blocking **muscarinic** receptors – a type of acetylcholine receptor concentrated in the brain, intestine, heart, smooth muscle and glands. The effects of muscarinic receptors include promotion of salivation and secretions in the airways, increase in intestinal movements and slowing of heart rate.

Curare

Curare is a plant extract that some S. American Indians use to poison their arrows and blow-darts. It is used during surgery as a muscle relaxant.

Mode of action

Curare blocks **nicotinic** receptors – another type of acetylcholine receptor found at the **neuromuscular junction** of skeletal muscle. This prevents stimulation of the muscle, and results in paralysis. The drug kills by paralysing the muscles that enable breathing.

Nicotine

Nicotine is an alkaloid substance found in the leaves of the tobacco plant. It is a drug used socially to provide a sense of well-being. However, it is also responsible for more damage to health in the UK than all other drugs (including alcohol) put together (pages 45 and 74).

Mode of action

Nicotine mimics the effect of the neurotransmitter acetylcholine. It acts directly on nicotinic receptors, producing its effects through stimulation of the central nervous system. Cigarette smoking delivers nicotine to the brain very efficiently. The drug is highly addictive. Many people who stop smoking initially experience withdrawal symptoms which include a craving for tobacco, irritability and loss of concentration.

Alcohol

Alcohol (ethanol), like nicotine, is a drug that is used socially. Alcoholic drink reduces inhibitions and gives people a sense of well-being, making it easier for them to socialise.

At low concentrations alcohol affects the frontal lobes of the brain. As more alcohol is consumed, further areas of the brain are affected, changing behaviour. Judgement, movement and then memory are impaired. Consumption of yet more alcohol may then affect brain centres vital for bodily functions. Heavy drinking over a long period leads to physical dependence, brain damage and liver disease (**cirrhosis**).

Mode of action

Alcohol affects the calcium channels of the pre-synaptic membrane. It inhibits the entry of calcium (Ca^{2+}) ions into the axon, and therefore prevents the release of neurotransmitter. As a result, the production of nerve impulses is reduced. Alcohol also stimulates release of the amino acid γ-**aminobutyric acid (GABA)** which inhibits the production of nerve impulses. These effects give alcohol its depressant action.

Heavy consumption of alcohol seems to increase the number of calcium channels, so that when alcohol is withdrawn transmitter release is abnormally high. The resulting overproduction of nerve impulses may contribute to the effects of withdrawal. Symptoms range from a 'hangover' to epileptic fits and even delirium tremens where the person becomes confused, agitated and suffers from hallucinations.

Caffeine

Caffeine is found in many different plants. The most common sources in the diet are coffee, tea and chocolate. Caffeine increases alertness and the ability to think clearly. Withdrawal effects may occur following high consumption of caffeine, including anxiety, irritability and muscle pains.

Mode of action

Caffeine stimulates the release of neurotransmitter from the pre-synaptic membrane. Increased activity of the brain produces the effects described.

Medical genetics

Our genetic make-up (**genotype**) contributes to many common diseases, for example our vulnerability to diabetes and heart disease. Environmental factors, however, also have their effect. Knowing about the genetic contribution to our vulnerability to disease helps us to avoid problems by taking account of the environmental factors within our control. In the cases of diabetes and heart disease for example, a sensible diet helps increase our chances of reaching a ripe old age (page 68).

Medical genetics establishes the genetic basis of disease and guides the treatment of people with genetic disorders. It also provides the data which inform potential parents about the genetic risks of starting a family.

Any prospective or expectant parents who have reason to be worried about genetic disorders that their future children might inherit can receive genetic counselling (page 99). During genetic counselling, statistical evidence and results from amniocentesis, chorionic villus sampling (page 90) or other techniques are discussed by a trained genetic counsellor with the couple concerned. The counselling helps couples make informed choices about whether to start a family if there is a chance of them having children with genetic disorders. It also helps expectant mothers and their partners to decide whether to continue with a pregnancy when they know their baby has a genetic disorder.

11.1 Techniques

Before continuing you need to remember that:
- Genes are carried on chromosomes which form pairs during meiosis. The two chromosomes of a pair are called **homologous chromosomes**.
- A gene is a length of DNA that codes for a particular protein, which is the gene product. We say that the gene **expresses** the product.
- Any particular characteristic (e.g. an enzyme, hormone, etc.) is controlled by pairs of genes called **alleles**.

- A pair of alleles may be the same (**homozygous**) or different (**heterozygous**).
- A **dominant** allele masks the effect of its **recessive** partner.

Estimates suggest that there are 3000 million base pairs in the chromosomes of a human cell. Laboratories in the USA, Europe and Japan are working to locate the position of individual genes on the chromosomes and to sequence the base pairs of each gene. The project is run by the **Human Genome Organisation (HUGO)**. It is the largest undertaking ever in the history of biological research.

Genetic defects are the cause of around 4000 inherited diseases. Understanding the genetic basis of disease comes down to locating and isolating the genes responsible on particular chromosomes, sequencing them, and identifying the abnormalities that cause different disorders.

Karyotyping (page 91) determines the number, size and shape of chromosomes, and identifies homologous pairs. Some genetic diseases caused by abnormalities in the number of chromosomes can be detected in the karyotype. For example, Down's syndrome and abnormal combinations of the X and Y chromosomes are caused by **non-disjunction** – a defect of cell division where homologous chromosomes or their **chromatids** fail to separate. Fig. 11.1 shows the result of the non-disjunction that causes Down's syndrome.

Other chromosomal abnormalities are made visible in a karyotype through the use of specific reagents which stain chromosomes to reveal banding patterns. Each band represents the position of dozens of genes. **Deletions** (the loss of part of a chromosome) and **translocations** (the transfer and incorporation of the deleted part of a chromosome into another non-homologous chromosome) produce visible abnormalities in the banding patterns of chromosomes. The discrepancies help to locate

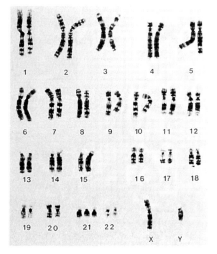

Figure 11.1   Karyotype of a man with Down's syndrome (compare with fig. 9.5).

genetic defects which cause disease. For example, some cases of Down's syndrome may result from a translocation in the chromosomes of one of the parents. The affected person has the third chromosome 21 attached to another chromosome – usually chromosome 14. Although the individual has only 46 chromosomes, he or she has the functional equivalent of a third chromosome 21. In young children, a deletion on chromosome 11 is associated with a type of cancer of the kidney called **Wilms tumour**. Another condition called **aniridia** (the congenital absence of the iris of the eye) is also associated with the same deletion. Wilm's tumour need not develop just because a child has the deletion on chromosome 11, but if he or she has aniridia *and* the deletion, then the risk is high. Detection of both defects means that treatment for Wilms' tumour can begin at an early stage, improving the chances of a successful outcome.

Linkage studies help locate the position of disease-causing genes. **DNA markers** which can be identified and which lie close enough to the genes of interest so that marker and gene remain together (linked) at cell division, are used to track disease genes through families. By studying affected and unaffected members of a family with a 'problem' gene, the likelihood of children inheriting the disorder can be predicted with some accuracy. However, there is nearly always a margin of error because of the risk that marker and gene will separate through recombination at cell division. The closer together the marker and gene, the less likely it is that separation will occur, so the more accurate will be the genetic prediction.

Analysing DNA

In 1969, bacterial enzymes were discovered that were able to recognise and cut out specific DNA sequences from long strands of DNA. This discovery was crucial to the development of techniques for the analysis of human DNA. Called **restriction enzymes**, each one recognises a particular DNA sequence (**recognition site**) and chops up strands of DNA into fragments called **restriction fragment length polymorphisms – RFLPs** or 'rif-lips' for short. The fragments can be arranged in order by **electrophoresis** and other techniques which sort substances according to size. The pattern of fragments is constant in an individual but varies between people because of differences in non-coding DNA sequences between genes (page 125).

DNA probes were another important step in the development of techniques for the analysis of DNA. Each one is a single strand of DNA used to detect complementary sequences in the fragments of DNA (RFLPs) produced by restriction enzymes. A probe binds to the DNA fragment that has a matching DNA sequence. The binding process is called DNA **hybridisation**. The probe may correspond to the gene under study and therefore locate its position directly. Alternatively, DNA nearby may be marked by the probe, locating a site linked to the gene of interest.

Radiolabelling the probe with phosphorus-32 identifies the hybridised fragments as bands on an **autoradiograph** which provides visible patterns for analysis.

Molecular biology of genetic diseases

The analysis of RFLPs was first used to diagnose sickle-cell anaemia (page 13). DNA from people with normal haemoglobin and from people with sickle-cell anaemia was cut into RFLPs using a restriction enzyme called *Hpa*1. A radioactive probe for the gene expressing the component of the haemoglobin molecule affected by sickle-cell anaemia was added to the RFLPs. The probe hybridised with a restriction fragment containing the normal haemoglobin gene consisting of either 7000 or 7600 base pairs. However, in the majority of sickle-cell cases, the probe hybridised with a restriction fragment of around 13 000 base pairs. Autoradiography and electrophoresis show the difference, which is due to the mutation causing sickle-cell anaemia altering the *Hpa*1 recognition sequence on the gene. Figure 11.2 shows the basis of the test.

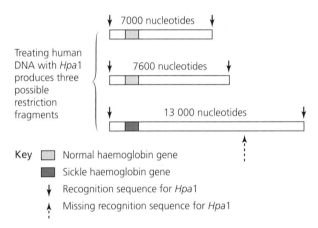

Figure 11.2 Using RFLPs to detect the presence of the sickle-cell gene. Combining the mixture of RFLPs with a probe for the haemoglobin gene produces probe–RFLP hybrids of different lengths that can be sorted for size. Detection of the probe–RFLP hybrid which is 13 000 nucleotides long is a diagnosis for the presence of the sickle haemoglobin gene.

Fetal haemophilia can be diagnosed by testing for fetal factor VIII (page 35) but only after 20 weeks of pregnancy. Earlier diagnosis is now possible using RFLPs to detect mutations in the gene expressing factor VIII. The test identifies women who are carriers of the disease, and also detects fetal haemophilia at a very early stage of pregnancy.

The development of RFLPs, gene probes and other molecular techniques for the detection of abnormal genes has revolutionised medical genetics. The diagnosis of genetic disease in fetuses, and the detection of parents' potential for passing on genetic disorders, provide the basic data for detailed and effective genetic counselling (page 99).

11.2 Inheritance of genetic disorders

Genes for genetic disorders are carried either on the sex chromosomes (X and Y) or on the other chromosomes (called the **autosomes**). Autosomal disorders have an equal chance of affecting males or females. Defective genes carried on the X chromosome are said to be **X-linked** and usually affect only males.

Most of us carry some defective genes. Fortunately, we usually have a normal copy of the allele which masks the effect of its abnormal recessive partner. However, if the defective allele is dominant or a person inherits two copies of a defective recessive allele (one from each parent) then the affected individual inherits the disorder. The various possibilities have a clear pattern of Mendelian inheritance (dominant, recessive or X-linked) so that the risk of someone inheriting a particular disorder can be predicted.

X-linked diseases

The allele responsible for haemophilia is recessive and located on the X chromosome. Although women may carry the defective allele on one of the X chromosomes, they do not usually suffer from haemophilia because the normal allele on the other X chromosome is dominant. The dominant allele masks the effect of its recessive partner and ensures that enough factor VIII is made for normal blood clotting to take place. A woman who has the recessive allele on one of the X chromosomes is called a **carrier**. Although she does not suffer from the disease, she is able to pass it on to her children. For a woman to have haemophilia, she would have had to receive the recessive allele from both her mother and her father. Since the recessive allele is rare, this only happens very occasionally.

Men have one X chromosome and one Y chromosome. The Y chromosome does not carry as many genes as the X chromosome. If a man inherits the recessive allele for haemophilia on the X chromosome, there is no dominant allele on the Y chromosome to mask the effect of its recessive partner. No factor VIII is produced and the man suffers from haemophilia.

Muscular dystrophy is another X-linked disorder. Affected muscle fibres deteriorate and the muscles progressively waste away to be replaced by fatty tissue. Females are unaffected but may be carriers of the defective gene. Mothers who are carriers can pass on the disease to their sons. Duchenne muscular dystrophy is the most common form of the disease, affecting around 1 in 3000 boys.

Families affected with defective genes cannot be counselled until individual carriers have been identified. Only then is it possible to draw up a **pedigree chart** showing genetic data about related individuals. Pedigree charts are used to predict the pattern of inherited disorders in future generations.

Autosomal recessive disorders

Cystic fibrosis (CF) is the most common autosomal recessive disorder in people of Northern European descent. About 1 in 20 of the population is a carrier, and in the UK one child in 2000 is born with the disorder. The defect has been identified as a mutation on chromosome 7 of an allele called the **cystic fibrosis transmembrane conductance regulator gene (CFTR)**. The normal allele encodes a polypeptide which functions as a channel for the movement of chloride ions (CI⁻) across the cell membrane. The commonest mutation involves deletion of the codon specifying the amino acid phenylalanine at position 508 in the polypeptide chain and accounts for over 70% of all CFTR mutations in Northern Europeans. The deletion affects membrane chloride channels and the movement of chloride ions, producing symptoms that include the overproduction of mucus in the lungs. Sufferers need physiotherapy every day to clear the mucus from the lungs.

As the allele is recessive, a person suffering from CF must have inherited two defective alleles (the homozygous condition) – one from each parent. Figure 11.3 charts the possibilities. Sickle-cell anaemia (page 13) shows a similar pattern of inheritance.

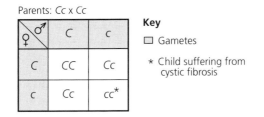

Parents: Cc x Cc

Key
☐ Gametes

* Child suffering from cystic fibrosis

Figure 11.3   Pattern of inheritance of cystic fibrosis.

Phenylketonuria is one of the best studied examples of a genetic disorder which causes an inborn error of metabolism. A mutation on chromosome 12 of the gene that normally encodes for **phenylalanine hydroxylase** prevents production of the enzyme. Phenylalanine and its by-products accumulate in the blood and urine, damaging cells of the nervous system and causing seizures and severe mental retardation.

Like other autosomal recessive diseases, a person with phenylketonuria must have inherited a defective allele from each parent (the homozygous condition). About 1 in 15 000 babies suffers from the problem, but early identification (in the fetus or at birth) allows the baby's diet to be managed, which effectively prevents damage. Treatment consists of special foods which limit the intake of phenylalanine to only that essential for normal growth.

Autosomal dominant disorders

Huntington's chorea is the best known autosomal dominant disorder. It is caused by mutation of an allele on chromosome 4. The condition is characterised by the progressive development of dementia and involuntary muscular movements. The age of onset of symptoms is on average 35 years, with a life expectancy thereafter of about 15 years. The majority of those affected can have children before being aware of their own condition.

Predictive testing for Huntington's chorea uses probe-detected RFLPs generated by cutting DNA with the restriction enzyme *Hind*III. DNA fragments marking the defective gene can be tracked through affected families.

Because it is dominant, only one allele is needed to cause Huntington's chorea. Both sexes can be equally affected at a frequency of around 5 in 100 000. Figure 11.4 shows that affected people are heterozygous (compare with the homozygous condition required for autosomal recessive disorders), although theoretically two heterozygous parents could produce a homozygous child. However, the effect would probably be lethal, and in any case Huntington's gene is so rare that it is unlikely to occur in the homozygous condition.

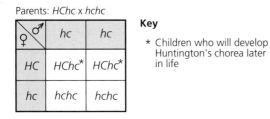

Parents: *HChc* x *hchc*

Key

* Children who will develop Huntington's chorea later in life

Figure 11.4   Pattern of inheritance of Huntington's chorea.

Achondroplasia (dwarfism due to short limbs) is another common disorder caused by a dominant allele. Although achondroplastic dwarfs are less likely to have children than other people, the condition regularly reappears because the gene involved mutates frequently.

Gene therapy

Gene therapy aims to add normal genes to a person's faulty genotype or repair faulty genes themselves. Before gene therapy can begin, DNA analysis is used to identify the defect. However, although transfer of functioning genes is theoretically possible, and figure 11.5 outlines a possible approach, many problems remain to be overcome.

To be successful, the donor gene should be stable once incorporated into the host's genotype, and produce adequate amounts of product (hormone, enzyme, etc.) in a controlled manner within the target cells. Also, insertion of a donor gene may disrupt a normal host gene, replacing one genetic disorder with another or possibly increasing the chance of cancer. These risks would be even more alarming were they to occur in eggs and sperm, because the problems would then be inherited by future generations.

In countries where research on gene therapy is in progress, the risks of new treatments have led to a number of recommendations. For the time being, gene therapy in the UK is restricted to the treatment of life-threatening conditions for which there is no alternative approach. Also, techniques are applied to body cells only and not to eggs and sperm. Possible risks that might result from genetic modifications will therefore not be inherited. The recommendations have cleared the way for treatments involving gene therapy to begin.

Attempts to cure cystic fibrosis (page 122) using gene therapy have met with mixed success. One approach incorporates healthy genes into fatty droplets called **liposomes** which are then sprayed as a fine aerosol deep into the lungs. Fusion of the liposomes with cells lining the patient's

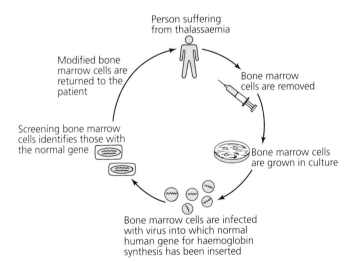

Figure 11.5 Thalassaemia is an important inherited cause of anaemia due to a deficiency in haemoglobin synthesis. Using gene therapy, the normal human gene for haemoglobin synthesis is inserted into a virus which is then used to infect a culture of bone marrow cells taken from the patient. Screening the bone marrow cells identifies the cells with the normal haemoglobin gene inserted. These modified cells are returned to the patient. (Adapted from Helen M. Kingston, 1994, *ABC of Clinical Genetics*, 2nd ed., BMJ Publishing Group.)

alveoli should enable the healthy genes to enter the cells and do their work. However gene transfer from liposomes to cells is not always successful, and when it does occur any beneficial effects are short lived. Work continues to improve the reliability of gene transfer and long-term effectiveness of the treatment.

A very rare condition called **severe combined immunodeficiency (SCID)** has been the subject of gene therapy treatment in the USA and UK. The disorder is caused by the failure of a gene to produce **adenosine deaminase (ADA)**. Without the enzyme, toxins which destroy the white blood cells accumulate in the blood. As a result the body is unable to fight infections which a healthy immune system would otherwise normally destroy. In gene therapy trials, white blood cells were taken from a patient and treated with a virus genetically engineered to carry a healthy copy of the ADA gene. The virus introduced the healthy gene into the white blood cells which were then returned to the patient's bloodstream. The hope was that the modified white blood cells would make ADA and establish the conditions for a functioning immune system. In some patients modified cells survived for as long as six months and their health improved. However, long-term the effectiveness of the treatment remains in doubt.

The CF and SCID trials highlight some of the difficulties encountered when using gene therapy. Fear of unknown effects on healthy genes and the risks of passing on modified genes to future generations are just a few of the concerns which make doctors and scientists cautious about the treatment. Looking to the future, recent developments pose serious ethical questions. Should we allow normal human characteristics to be changed by gene therapy? Who should receive treatment first – the young who are seriously ill or the old on the verge of death? Risks and benefits need thorough discussion if we are to make progress safely and for the benefit of all of society.

11.3 Genetic fingerprinting

Between 20 and 30% of human DNA is made up of regions of short, highly repetitive sequences called **simple-sequence DNA**. Each sequence is typically 5 to 10 base pairs in length. Simple-sequence DNA is thought to be vital to chromosome structure. For example, the tips of human chromosomes each consist of a 'cap' of the repeated simple sequence TTAGGG, 1500 to 6000 base pairs in length.

The number of repeated units in each region of simple-sequence DNA varies from person to person and is as unique to the individual as his or her fingerprints. This uniqueness is the basis for genetic fingerprinting, which can help to identify criminals in cases where the criminal's body cells are left at the scene of the crime. Regions of simple-sequence DNA are cut from the biological evidence (traces of blood or semen, for example) with appropriate restriction enzymes, separated by length using eletrophoresis, identified by a radioactively labelled probe and visualised on an autoradiograph. The end result looks like a bar code, and is unique to the criminal in question. Suspects may be genetically fingerprinted and their bar codes compared with the bar code obtained from the evidence (figure 11.6). Matching bar codes (from suspect and evidence) identify the criminal, virtually beyond reasonable doubt. Except in the case of identical twins, the chance of two people having the same number of repeat sequences in regions of simple-sequence DNA are millions to one against.

Often, only traces of biological evidence are found at the scene of a crime. A technique of gene amplification called **polymerase chain reaction (PCR)** can take a minute segment of DNA and, within hours, synthesise millions of copies. PCR provides sufficient material to obtain DNA fingerprints from the slightest piece of evidence – the root of a single hair will do. PCR also has medical value. It can be used to speed up the diagnosis of genetic disease in the fetus, allowing early decisions to be made about the progress of the pregnancy. The safety of the mother and the fetus is also improved because only a small amount of material is required for amplication before testing.

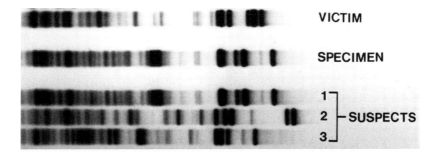

Figure 11.6 DNA fingerprints from a rape victim, the semen specimen and three suspects. Which suspect matches the specimen?

11.4 Genetics of tissue compatibility

Cell membranes carry histocompatibility antigens (abbreviated to HLA in humans), which are responsible for tissue rejection following transplant surgery (page 29). The genes coding for HLA form four closely linked clusters on chromosome 6: *HLA-A*, *HLA-B*, *HLA-C* and *HLA-D*. With only four gene clusters, how is it possible for each person to have a practically unique set of HLA antigens? Table 11.1 provides an answer. Notice that each gene cluster consists of a number of alleles (page 117). The number of possible genotypes for each cluster can be calculated as:

$$\frac{n\,(n+1)}{2}$$

where n is the number of alleles in the cluster. For example, for *HLA-A*:

$$\text{number of possible genotypes} \quad = \quad \frac{26\,(26+1)}{2} \quad = \quad 351$$

Calculating the number of possible genotypes for each of the other gene clusters and multiplying the four numbers together shows that billions of different genotypes are possible. No wonder nearly everyone has a unique set of HLA antigens.

The figures illustrate the size of the task facing scientists trying to match donor organs to recipients who need transplant surgery. Tissue typing tries to achieve as close a match as possible (page 29).

Table 11.1. The number of alleles in each *HLA* cluster

Gene cluster	Number of alleles
HLA-A	26
HLA-B	35
HLA-C	14
HLA-D	87

11.5 Environmental factors linked to cancer

Various factors in the environment may interfere with normal cells. For example, different substances (called **carcinogens**) in cigarette smoke and foods damage genes and can cause cancer. So too can viruses, radiation and overexposure to sunlight. Faulty genes are associated with cancer of the bladder, bowel, breast and ovary. However, someone who has these faulty genes will not necessarily develop cancer – several different triggers are probably involved.

Smoking

In the UK, approximately 50 000 deaths from cancer each year are linked to smoking, making tobacco the single most important cause of cancer (especially lung cancer). The risk of developing cancer is reduced by stopping smoking, and decreases substantially after five years of giving up. Unburnt tobacco contains at least 2500 chemicals. Of these substances, different forms of N-nitrosoamines and metal compounds have been identified as carcinogens. To understand their effects we must first understand **oncogenes** and **tumour suppressor genes**.

Oncogenes are formed as a result of mutations that increase the activity of genes which stimulate cell division. In their normal state, these genes control cell division such that it stops when enough cells have been made to perform a particular task – healing a cut, for example (page 35). When mutations convert the genes to oncogenes, cell division runs out of control. As a result, cells proliferate contributing to the development of cancer. The most common oncogenes involved with cancer (25% of lung cancer) are the *ras* oncogenes, and these can be induced by the carcinogens in cigarette smoke.

Tumour suppressor genes inhibit cell division, and tobacco carcinogens may lead to mutations which cause their loss or inactivation. Again, cell division runs out of control. The tumour suppressor gene called *p53* is most frequently involved.

Oncogenes and the mutation of tumour suppressor genes increase cell division and the loss of growth control. The result – cancers, of which lung cancer is the most common (table 1.2).

Radiation

Different human activities generate various forms of radiation. Some of these, including radio waves for communication, microwaves for cooking and radar for navigation, are **non-ionising.** Emissions from radioactive substances, on the other hand, are **ionising** radiations. They can change (damage) molecules, including DNA, by stripping electrons from matter exposed to them (ionisation). Radioactive materials in the Earth's crust and cosmic rays from space are sources of the environment's **background radiation** to which all living things are exposed. Background radiation is, in part, responsible for the changes in the structure of DNA (mutations) that occur in all organisms.

Radiation may cause mutations by damaging DNA *directly*, or by generating highly active components of molecules called **free radicals** which cause the damage *indirectly*. Free radicals are formed, for example, by the action of radiation on water molecules.

The development of nuclear technologies has increased our exposure to radiation over and above the background count. Fallout from the testing of nuclear weapons, the use of X-rays for medical purposes and dumping radioactive waste from nuclear power stations combine to increase mutation rates. In particular, there are unanswered questions about the safety of nuclear power stations. Different investigations have suggested that the incidence of **leukaemia** (a cancer of the white blood cells) in children living near to nuclear installations may be greater than would be expected normally. For example, a recent study identified seven cases of childhood leukaemia in the population living near to the Sellafield nuclear installation when an average of less than one case would have been expected. Leukaemia can be caused by ionising radiation.

Leukaemia clusters have also been identified around the Dounreay nuclear research establishment in Scotland, and the nuclear weapons sites of Aldermaston and Burghfield. Confirming that radioactive discharges from these sites are the *cause* of the clusters is difficult to establish. Evidence suggests that men working at the Sellafield site are more likely to father children who develop leukaemia, but similar assessment at Dounreay neither proved nor disproved the link.

To date, the evidence is inconclusive. However, it suggests that there is an *association* (page 57) between exposure to low levels of radiation in excess of background and the development of leukaemia – either through the direct exposure of children or through chromosome defects in people who work in the nuclear industry and who then have children. Whatever the outcome of further investigations, the message is clear: exposure to excess levels of radiation should be kept as low as possible. Any increase will increase the mutation rate, with the possibility of harmful effects on people's health.

Malignant **melanoma** of the skin is a cancer arising from the **melanocytes** (pigment-producing cells) in the skin. In recent years the occurrence of melanoma worldwide has increased significantly (more than 6% per year in England and Wales). The disease is more common in fair-skinned people than in dark-skinned people, and is more common in people who are freckled, have blue eyes and fair hair. Overexposure to sunlight (e.g. during early childhood or on holidays) seems to be the major risk factor. Treatment of melanoma is usually by surgical removal of the growth, and the prospects of cure are good providing metastasis (page 18) has not occurred. However, metastasis is rapid, so early detection is important.

Nonmelanoma skin cancers are also caused by overexposure to sunlight. They are common but rarely lethal because metastasis is slow. Treatment is by surgery or radiotherapy.

Ultraviolet (UV) radiation is the part of the sun's electromagnetic spectrum that causes the damage. Table 11.2 shows the different components of UV and their effects on the skin. Notice that UVB is a major risk factor causing melanoma. However, uncertainties about the hazards of exposure to UVA suggest that UVA sun-beds to develop a winter tan should be used with caution. Their increasing availability for home use is a cause for some concern among scientists and doctors worried about trends in the occurrence of skin cancers.

UV radiation striking skin cells generates free radicals which may damage DNA in the nucleus – perhaps especially the *p53* suppressor gene

Table 11.2. Components of UV and their effects on the skin

UV component	Effect on skin
UVA	Darkens pigment in the skin and causes a tan to develop. Does not burn but may damage deeper levels of the skin.
UVB	Major risk factor for melanoma. Burns the skin.
UVC	Very damaging to the skin, but is mostly screened out by the ozone layer.

and *ras* oncogenes (page 127). Normally DNA repair systems in the cells swing into action and correct the damage – a process called **unscheduled DNA repair**. However, if DNA repair does not occur in melanocytes then the resulting abnormal DNA synthesis forms more abnormal melanocytes. A clone of malignant melanoma cells then develops. UV radiation also reduces the effectiveness of the immune system (chapter 2). This immunosuppression makes it less likely that the body will recognise the malignant melanocytes and eliminate them.

Protection
Clothes and a broad-brimmed hat protect the body from overexposure to the sun. **Sunscreen** preparations smeared over bare skin also help. They reduce burning effects and may help prevent skin cancer by filtering UV, mainly in the UVB range.

Each sunscreen preparation has a **sun protection factor (SPF)** which gives an idea of how much longer it takes for sunburn to occur compared with no sunscreen. For example, with factor 10, a person can spend ten times longer in the sun than if they were unprotected before burning. Choice of sunscreen depends on skin type and the associated risk of burning. At least factor 10 is recommended for people with fair skin.

T W E L V E

Biotechnology and medicine

Date: 15 October 1980. *Place*: New York Stock Exchange. The launch of a small company called Genentech sparked frenetic business, driving up its share price from $35 to $89 within the first 20 minutes of trading. At the end of the day, each Genentech share was worth $71.25. Why was there so much interest in a small four-year-old Californian company specialising in **genetic engineering**?

Two years previously, scientists at Genentech had isolated the genes that code for the A and B polypeptide chains of human insulin, spliced them into a loop of bacterial DNA called a **plasmid** and inserted the modified plasmid into the bacterium *Escherichia coli*. They had achieved what previously had seemed impossible, but by today's standards is commonplace. An organism (*E. coli*) had been genetically engineered to produce a medicine (the hormone insulin used to treat diabetes) with a worldwide market worth many hundreds of millions of dollars a year. Before then, insulin could only be obtained from slaughtered cattle and pigs. It was expensive to produce and in limited supply. Also, the chemical structure of animal insulin is different from human insulin; some diabetics react allergically to it. Genentech's achievement seemed to open the way to the large-scale production of medicines which were reliable, cheap and, in the case of insulin, more suitable for the human patient. No wonder the New York Stock Exchange was frantic on that October day – the future promised not only medical progress but also unrivalled profits!

12.1 What is biotechnology and genetic engineering?

Biotechnology and genetic engineering are often thought of as one and the same thing. However, they are not. Biotechnology uses microorganisms (viruses, bacteria and fungi), plant cells and animal cells on a large scale for the production of commercially important products. Its processes have a long history. The use of moulds to make cheese and bacteria to make vinegar, are early examples. For thousands of years, yeast has been exploited to make bread, beer and wine.

The modern meaning of biotechnology was established in the 1960s. At that time, the way to increase productivity was to select mutant organisms which made more of the desired product. The procedures were costly in time and money, and often unreliable. In the 1970s scientists developed techniques (page 117) which allowed us to manipulate genes to our advantage. Genetic engineering had come of age, and its techniques changed biotechnology for ever. Because of genetic engineering, it is now possible to create organisms with specific genetic characteristics for producing medicines, foods and a range of industrial chemicals.

12.2 Genetically engineered hormones

Hormones are chemicals produced by the endocrine glands and released into the bloodstream. They regulate the body's activities. For example, different hormones, of which insulin is one, regulate the level of glucose in the blood by balancing the glucose-producing and glucose-using processes of the body. Insulin decreases the level of glucose in the blood

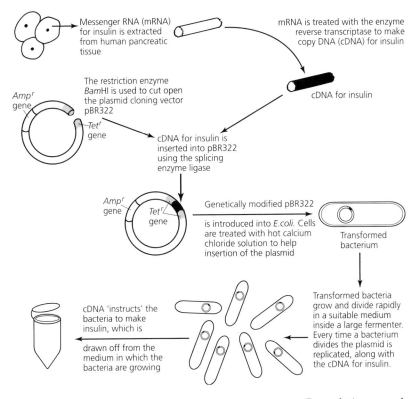

Figure 12.1 Producing insulin using genetic engineering. (For techniques used to genetically engineer the pBR322 plasmid, see chapter 11.)

by promoting the conversion of glucose into glycogen which is stored in the liver.

If the body does not produce enough insulin then a condition called **diabetes mellitus** occurs. The glucose level in the blood becomes dangerously high and glucose is excreted in the urine. A simple test for glucose in the urine can identify a person who is diabetic. In severe cases, diabetics are taught to inject themselves regularly with insulin to lower their blood glucose levels.

Figure 12.1 shows one way in which genetic engineering is used to make insulin. The human insulin gene is isolated and inserted into the plasmid cloning vector called pBR322, which in turn is inserted into the bacterium *Escherichia coli*. Notice that pBR322 carries two genes for resistance to antibiotics: one for resistance to tetracycline (*Tet*^{r}) and the other to ampicillin (*Amp*^{r}). Before insertion of the insulin gene, the plasmid's DNA loop is cut by the restriction enzyme (page 117) called *Bam*HI. Its recognition site (page 117) lies within the *Tet*^{r} gene. When the insulin gene is inserted into the recognition site, the *Tet*^{r} gene no longer functions properly. So, the *E. coli* which take up the engineered vector (**transformation**) are sensitive to tetracycline. Resistance to ampicillin, however, is unaffected because the *Amp*^{r} gene is intact.

Plasmids are self-replicating closed loops of DNA found in virtually all types of bacteria. **F plasmids** transfer from one cell to another. **R plasmids** code for resistance to antibiotics. Because they are self-replicating (i.e. produce clones of identical DNA) and transfer from cell to cell, plasmids are ideal vehicles (**cloning vectors**) for carrying foreign DNA into cells. In practice, however, not all plasmids are suitable cloning vectors, and those that are must be modified for the task.

The resistance genes are important when it comes to identifying the transformed bacteria colonies. Only transformed cells and 'normal' cells are able to grow on an agar plate containing ampicillin, because both types of cell are resistant to the antibiotic. All of the other combinations produced in the transformation process perish.

To pin-point colonies of *E. coli* making insulin, a membrane to which insulin antibodies are attached is lowered onto the agar–ampicillin plate on which mixed colonies are growing. Insulin molecules from the transformed cells attach to the membrane, which is transferred to a plate covered with radioactively labelled insulin antibodies. The antibody–insulin complex on the membrane picks up the labelled antibodies, and the membrane with its antibody–insulin–radioactive antibody combinations is placed over a photographic film. The resulting autoradiograph (page 120) maps the position of the insulin-manufacturing (i.e. transformed) colonies of bacteria. Individual cultures are established from these colonies and scaled up for commercial production of the hormone.

In the production of genetically engineered insulin, the gene inserted into the pBR322 plasmid is not actually for insulin but for **pro-insulin** which consists of a C polypeptide chain attached to the A and B chains. Pro-insulin is the inactive precursor of insulin. In production, pro-insulin is extracted and the C chain removed to form mature insulin.

Other genetically engineered hormones, including **human growth hormone (hGH)** and **calcitonin** (the hormone that controls the absorption of calcium into bones), are produced by methods similar to those for producing insulin. At one time, hGH was extracted from the pituitary glands of dead people. However, it was not possible to produce a completely pure product and there was a risk of transmitting the virus that causes the degenerative brain disorder **Creutzfeldt–Jacob** disease to patients receiving hormone treatment. Producing hGH from genetically engineered bacteria has eliminated the risk.

Apart from overcoming the problem of transmitting diseases in impure products, genetic engineering and biotechnology make available much larger quantities of hormones and other substances for the treatment of disease. In the case of hGH, growing 600 litres of genetically engineered bacteria produces as much hormone as 40 000 human pituitary glands. With the availability of large quantities of hGH, its use in the treatment of diseases other than **pituitary dwarfism** (cf. achondroplasia, page 123) is possible. Osteoporosis (page 18) and the healing of wounds, burns and broken bones may benefit from treatment with hGH.

12.3 Biosensors

An antibody will attach itself only to a particular antigen (page 22); an enzyme will catalyse only a particular reaction or group of reactions. **Biosensors** use the sensitivity of these reactions and microelectronic circuits to detect minute amounts of chemicals. In the future, biosensors will help scientists to diagnose disease and monitor pollution in the environment.

Immobilised enzymes are at the biological heart of different types of biosensor. For example, immobilised glucose oxidase is a vital part of the biosensor shown in figure 12.2. The enzyme catalyses the reaction:

$$C_6H_{12}O_6 + O_2 + H_2O \xrightarrow{\text{glucose oxidase}} \text{gluconic acid} + H_2O_2$$

glucose   oxygen   water   hydrogen peroxide

Key

$\circ_\circ$ Glucose molecules (the substrate to be detected)

P Product (gluconic acid) of interaction between substrate (glucose) and immobilised enzyme (glucose oxidase)

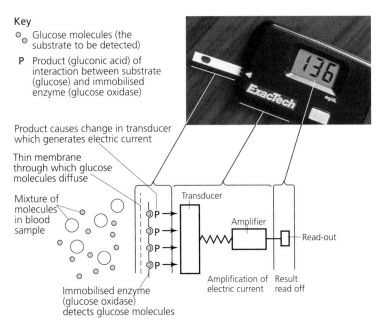

Product causes change in transducer which generates electric current

Thin membrane through which glucose molecules diffuse

Mixture of molecules in blood sample

Transducer

Amplifier

Read-out

Immobilised enzyme (glucose oxidase) detects glucose molecules

Amplification of electric current

Result read off

Figure 12.2 How a biosensor works. The blood sample, obtained using a sterile stab, activates the sensor.

The acid produced conducts an electrical current which is proportional to the amount of glucose in solution – an important measurement for someone suffering from diabetes. The glucose concentration in the blood is measured and converted into a digital read-out.

Immobilised enzymes

When an enzyme is added to the substances whose reaction it catalyses, it may be lost when the product is collected. Dilution also occurs, making it difficult to recover the enzyme when the extraction is complete. Recent developments in the manufacture of enzymes have overcome these problems. Various insoluble materials are used to bond to the enzyme, immobilising it. The enzyme can still catalyse reactions but remains attached to the insoluble support, and is not lost when the products are collected. Immobilised enzymes are easily recovered, not diluted and are often active at temperatures that would destroy the unprotected enzyme.

Some of the benefits of sensor technology come from the advantages of rapid analyses which identify drug and alcohol overdoses where treatment of the patient is urgent. Cumbersome and expensive laboratory equipment which may be too slow to be helpful in an emergency is no longer needed. Biosensors also allow more careful management of patients. For example, diabetic patients can self-test their blood glucose levels using the biosensor shown in figure 12.2. The tighter monitoring of glucose levels can help prevent some of the long-term complications associated with diabetes.

New manufacturing techniques are producing disposable biosensor strips, helping prevent the health risks associated with analyses of blood samples contaminated with, for example, HIV and hepatitis virus (page 6). Disposable sensors are available for the determination of blood glucose levels (diagnosis of diabetes), lactic acid levels (diagnosis of heart attack, page 39) and cholesterol (diagnosis of atherosclerosis).

12.4 Monoclonal antibodies

B lymphocytes produce millions of antibodies to defend the body from attack by bacteria, viruses, fungi and other potentially dangerous antigens (chapter 2). However, each molecule of antigen usually has several regions (each called an **epitope**) to which B cells respond by producing antibodies specific for each site. The mixture produced against an antigen's set of epitopes is called a **polyclonal antibody.**

It was recognised early on that antibodies could be used to prevent infections and diagnose diseases. However, the B cell response to each epitope of an antigen varies – some epitopes produce a stronger B cell response than other epitopes. Polyclonal antibody preparations, therefore, vary from batch to batch and are unreliable because at times some epitopes of a particular antigen strongly stimulate B cells to produce antibodies, whereas at other times B cells respond more actively to other epitopes. The problem can be overcome by fusing B cells that produce a particular antibody with a type of rapidly dividing lymphocyte cancer cell called a **myeloma**. The fused cells (called **hybridomas**) only produce the antibody required. Pure samples of antibodies produced in this way are called **monoclonal antibodies.**

Production technology

The first step in the production of hybrid cells which produce pure antibody against a particular antigen is to inoculate mice with the antigen in question. After several injections over a period of weeks, the mice are tested for an immune response to the antigen. If the results are positive, the mice are killed and their spleens (page 22) removed and processed to release cells, some of which are antibody-producing B cells.

Unfortunately, B cells do not grow in culture, though myelomas do. Fusion of normal B cells with myelomas produces hybridomas which grow in culture and produce the desired antibody. Cell fusion is promoted by mixing B cells and myelomas with polyethylene glycol. The fusion mixture is then cultured in a growth medium in which only B cell/myeloma hybrids (hybridomas) survive. The next stage isolates the hybrid cells producing the desired antibody. Once identified, the hybrid cells can be maintained more or less indefinitely in culture as a source of monoclonal antibody molecules that recognise the target antigen.

Applications of monoclonal antibodies

Monoclonal antibodies have a wide range of uses. For example, monoclonal antibodies may be used to treat cancer. Some types of cancer cell have proteins on their surface that are different from the proteins made by healthy cells. The cancer cell proteins are antigens that can be used to generate monoclonal antibodies using the methods just described. Because the monoclonal antibodies attach only to the proteins made by cancer cells, their combination with anti-cancer drugs makes it possible to target the cancer cells for destruction without affecting healthy cells (figure 12.3).

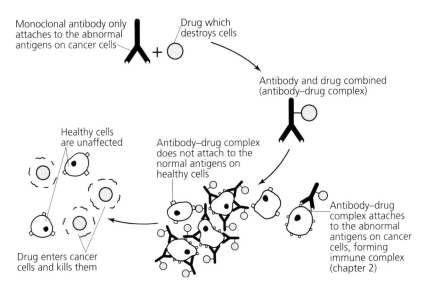

Figure 12.3 Using monoclonal antibodies to treat cancer.

Monoclonal antibodies have been put to other uses:
- The urine of pregnant women contains **human chorionic gonadotrophin (hCG)**. The hormone, produced by the placenta, can be detected using monoclonal antibodies as early as 12 days after fertilisation. The test kit consists of a dipstick impregnated with antibodies. The position of a coloured band after dipping the stick into a urine sample tells the woman whether or not she is pregnant. If hCG is present in the urine, the mollecules of

the hormone bind to the antibodies at the end of the dipstick. The hCG–antibody complex diffuses up the dipstick and meets a band of antibodies which also bind hCG. A colour change at this level shows that the woman is pregnant. If there is no hCG in the urine, antibodies alone diffuse up the dipstick to meet a second band of different antibodies. The antibodies bind together producing a colour change which shows that the woman is not pregnant.

- Monoclonal antibodies bind with poisons, inactivating them. Tetanus toxin and overdosage of digoxin (a drug used to treat heart disease) can be inactivated with different antibody types.
- The success of transplants depends on matching the tissues of donor and patient as nearly as possible. The closer the match, the less the chance of tissue rejection (page 29). Monoclonal anti-bodies, produced against the cell surface proteins of the donor's and patient's tissues, make tissue matching more accurate.

Developing different types of monoclonal antibody for medical and other uses is expensive. However, the potential for profit is considerable, resulting in new companies springing up in response to the demand.

12.5 Antibiotics

Penicillin was the first of a family of antibiotic drugs made by biotechnology. Today, hundreds of different antibiotics are used to combat diseases caused by bacteria, and many more substances with antibiotic activity have been discovered. However, most are too expensive for commercial production and/or have harmful side effects. Nevertheless, some have their uses outside medicine in research, agriculture and food production.

There are four groups of antibiotic:
- **Penicillins** – commercially produced penicillin is a mixture of compounds. The main component is penicillin G which can be converted into other forms, each with a slightly different activity. Penicillin G is broken down by stomach acid and can therefore be given by mouth as tablets or in syrup – something children may prefer! The range of penicillins allows medical staff to choose which type is the best for treating a particular disease. Choice also helps to combat the development of drug resistance.
- **Cephalosporins** – cephalosporins made by the mould *Cephalosporium* were discovered in 1948. All are active against a similar range of bacteria. Newer cephalosporins are effective against bacteria which have developed resistance to penicillin.

- **Tetracyclines** – tetracycline is made by the bacterium *Streptomyces aureofaciens*. Its various forms are active against a similar range of bacteria, although the development of widespread resistance has reduced their effectiveness. Tetracyclines bind to calcium and are deposited in growing bones and teeth. They therefore should not be given to children and pregnant women.
- **Erythromycins** – the activity range of erythromycin is similar to that of penicillin. It is therefore useful against bacteria resistant to penicillin or where the patient is allergic to penicillin.

Worldwide sales of antibiotics are worth billions of pounds each year. Some, like penicillin, destroy a limited number of species of bacteria. They are **narrow-spectrum** antibiotics. Others, such as tetracycline, are **broad-spectrum** antibiotics and act against a variety of species.

Penicillin production

At the beginning of the twentieth century, scientists noticed that laboratory cultures of bacteria did not grow on culture plates on which colonies of mould were also growing. Nobody followed up these observations until 1928, when the British bacteriologist Alexander Fleming working at St Mary's Hospital, London noticed that some of his bacteria cultures were contaminated with mould. Fleming identified the mould as *Penicillium notatum* and reasoned that it produced a substance which killed bacteria. He isolated the substance and called it penicillin.

Fleming thought that penicillin might help fight disease, but extracting it from the mould was difficult. There matters rested until 1938 when Howard Florey and Ernst Chain working at Oxford University made the commercial production of penicillin possible. The work moved to the USA where large-scale production techniques were developed, using 'cornsteep liquor' (a waste produced from the manufacture of starch from maize) as the nutrient solution for the growth of penicillin mould.

Penicillium notatum produces very little penicillin. *P. chrysogenum* yields more. Today, the massive demand for penicillin worldwide is met by the development of new, high-yielding strains. Yield can now be improved through genetic engineering and advances in the control of fermentation processes. One approach has been to isolate the gene for **isopenicillin N synthetase** from *P. chrysogenum*. The enzyme catalyses an important step in the synthesis of penicillin N – a key intermediate compound in the manufacture of penicillins (and also cephalosporins). Penicillins are produced in large containers called fermenters which hold up to 200 000 litres of nutrient/genetically engineered mould solution. At the end of the process the mould is filtered off and the penicillin extracted from solution by the addition of sodium or potassium compounds which promote the formation of penicillin crystals.

Index

SHREWSBURY COLLEGE
LONDON RD. LRC